Body Confidence
From the Inside Out

Body Confidence
From the Inside Out

by

Penny Plautz

Whole Person Associates
Duluth, Minnesota

Whole Person Associates
210 West Michigan
Duluth, MN 55802
1-800-247-6789

Body Confidence From the Inside Out

Printed in the United States of America.

Library of Congress Control Number: 2006929002

ISBN 1-57025-245-9
ISBN-13 978-1-57025-245-7

Dedication

For my grandmother, Idella Upton,
whose steady supply of letters over the years
taught me the magic of words.

Table of Contents

Acknowledgements   ix

Introduction   xi

How to Get the Most Out of This Book and Yourself   xv

Body Confidence Journal Pages   xxi

Part One

    What Happened?   1

    Start Where You Are   13

    Examine Your Expectations   27

    Explore Your Options   39

    Lighten Your Load   51

    Stretch Your Knowledge   63

    Feed Your Curiosity   79

    Build Your Personal Power   93

    Move Into Your Life   107

    Body Confidence in the Bedroom, Boardroom & Beyond   121

    Resource Central   135

Part Two

    Facilitating Body Confidence   147

    Planning Pages   159

About the Author   196

Acknowledgements

Like Body Confidence, a book does not come into being without inexhaustible enthusiasm and the unflinching support of many people. My sincerest thanks go to following people:

Idella Upton, my grandmother, who at 88 is fit as a fiddle and shows no signs of slowing down; she has believed in me ever since I learned to write.

My students, past and present, they are the real teachers; their courage, discipline, and beauty astounds me on a regular basis; go forth and blossom!

My Awesome Advisory Board, past and present: Philip Humbert, Mary Ertle, Mershon Neisner, Noah Rolland, Barbara Gormally, Linda Brakeall, Penney Pierce, and Suzanne Falter-Barns.

My fellow instructors, who are also part of my Awesome Advisory Board, and who gave me a place to teach in their clubs and studios: JoAnn Bishop, Jackie Camborde, Chip Conway, Lisa Gulotta, and Marce Miller.

My global R & D team, especially Terry Boyer, Maree Crosbie, Zafira Labadi, Vicky Vogel, Deborah Jessop, Eleonor Hellman, Ann McClain, Marvi Letey, Cathy Flum, Fran Trant, Caryl Fairbank, Betty Purkey, and Diane Borre.

My family, for helping me transform an old apartment into an exercise studio, and for supporting my creatively quirky lifestyle; special thanks to my mom, Nancy Plautz, for following me around the country in support of my work, and my sister, Kellie Larrabee, for always being there, ready to listen and support even with a full life of her own.

My Wellpower partner, Tom Bonow, for keeping us in business while I finished the book and devoting the "angel corner" of the office to this project.

The folks at Whole Person Associates, specifically my editor, Susan Rubendall, for her "book confidence" and help in getting this one into shape.

You, for trusting me to lead you to a place of Body Confidence.

Introduction

"How does one become a butterfly?" she asked.

"You must want to fly so much that you are willing to give up being a caterpillar."

Trina Paulus, *Hope for the Flowers*

Despite evidence to the contrary, an amazing thing happens when a woman ages. While the rest of the world may be writing her off as over the hill, past her prime, undesirable, invisible, or any number of euphemisms for women of a certain age, an inner feistiness festers. Inevitably this feistiness erupts in a fit of fearlessness, and most astonishingly, a carnal confidence unbeknownst to her at an earlier age emerges.

I did not know this when I was approaching forty. Consequently, panic set in. I feared my inner Frump Queen would usher herself in and take over the next decade. In a preemptive strike, I decided to write down everything I had learned about life, liberty, and the pursuit of happiness — at least as it pertained to my body. I considered it a manifesto for the woman who was never going to fit into a size six and refused to die trying. I could also rant about aging gracefully and living a courageously quirky life. If ever there was a time to shed the shame that shackled me to the insanity of a society obsessed with youth and physical perfection, it was now.

Yet without a compelling reason to record these convictions, I knew the zest I felt for my manifesto would pass as predictably as PMS. So I created an email course called Body Confidence and invited anyone with an Internet connection to join me.

Over 60 women and a few men from around the globe agreed to

participate in the first email course. It was a leap of faith for all involved. None of us knew what was in store. We just knew the idea of Body Confidence was worth exploring.

Part One of this book contains many of the original lessons and exercises that emerged from that course. Part Two offers you ways to incorporate these lessons in group settings, coaching, or therapeutic environments.

Most programs start by making changes on the outside that fail to spark an inner evolution. Body Confidence is the extreme makeover that begins within. It does not depend on the skills of plastic surgeons, personal trainers and chefs, psychiatrists and therapists, or makeup artists and beauticians for you to recognize your own beauty and power. It does not rely on thousands of viewers to validate your worth by witnessing your amazing results in a span of sixty minutes. And best of all, it doesn't cost a small fortune.

It does, however, depend on your willingness to show up, do the exercises, dig deep, be brave, tell the truth, act with integrity, hang in there when things get hard, and invest in a good pair of athletic shoes and a step counter. (A few fabulous exercise outfits will also work wonders.)

If you are reading this book, you are either at war with your body, have spent significant time in the trenches, or work with and care deeply about someone whose body is her battlefield. Some of you have waged this war for a lifetime. Others took up the fight after the birth of a child, a health crisis, a divorce, a death, a marriage, a career move, or other significant change.

It's time to call a cease-fire. In Body Confidence you are asked to surrender your weapons of mass distraction and allow yourself to experience peace. Having said that, I know you warriors will insist you cannot comfortably exist without your stockpile of ammunition. An excess of unused equipment such as dumbbells, jump ropes, boxing gloves, punching bags, stairclimbers, treadmills, balance balls, workout videos, energy bars, and digital scales does little more than create a shrine to Our Lady of Perpetual Guilt.

I'm not asking you to give up the stuff. I am asking you to give up the notion that all this stuff can instantly transform you into a sleeker, sexier, sassier sliver of your former self. If you cannot recognize your innate beauty, intelligence, and strength right now, no amount of outer transformation will be enough. You must begin from within, from a position of power and a place of self-respect. Confidence does not come from shaming, blaming, or shoulding.

So what exactly is "Body Confidence"?

It's being at home in your body. It's knowing you can respond to the physical and psychological demands you place on your body. It's fueling yourself with proper nutrition so you can perform at optimal levels. It's being able to interpret your body's feedback. It's an appreciation of your sensuality. It's a deep respect for the form that contains your remarkable spirit. It's feeling fabulous in the skin you're in regardless of your age, size, or perceived imperfections.

How is this approach different than others you may have tried before? Basically, Body Confidence starts with the premise that there is nothing wrong with you. Most programs assume the reason you want to change is because there is something dreadfully wrong with the way you are right now.

Believing things must be fixed, firmed, flattened, lost, lifted, liposuctioned, stretched, or strengthened before you can feel confident or comfortable in your body denies you the pleasure of being present in your body right now. If you don't like your body now, how will you make the leap to loving it when it's "perfect?"

By working through this book you will discover the thrill of becoming strong, flexible, and alive in your body. You will know the power and grace that come from belonging in your body. You will define what matters most to you and learn to live with that as your center of power.

And hopefully, you will surround yourself with others who support your transformation. You may even inspire theirs!

If you could have done this by yourself, you would have done it by now. It's not that you don't know how to reach your health and fitness goals. It's that you don't know how to stay motivated to maintain these goals. You may not yet realize that being healthy is its own reward — a reward you deserve to experience every day of your life.

You have an unlimited well of power within you. By accessing it, you will astound your skeptical self. You will put on your walking shoes and head out the door — even when conditions are less than ideal. You will be satisfied with two bites of chocolate cake instead of two pieces. You may still dread dressing-room mirrors during swimsuit season, but you will be proud of the person reflected back to you.

This is not a book about losing weight, imparting the Absolute Truth about nutrition, being able to run a marathon, and lift the equivalent of a Volkswagen Beetle. If any of the above occurs, consider it a bonus!

My primary intention is to help you become aware of the patterns, the people, the places, and the perspectives that have shaped your life and your body up to this point. Exposing these factors frees you to make different choices.

I have been a fitness professional for twenty years. I have seen what people sacrifice in the pursuit of physical perfection. I also know that "perfection" is, at best, elusive. And without Body Confidence to back it up, it means nothing.

I am thrilled to have you join me on this journey. I want to thank you in advance for your courage and commitment.

Now, let's get started!

How to Get the Most Out of
This Book and Yourself

There are as many ways to read this book as there are readers. As with most things, some ways work better than others. I will give you the benefit of my experience and let you decide how to proceed. Whether you are reading this on your own or as part of a group, these guidelines will help you get the most out of this book and yourself. Additional guidelines for facilitators are listed in Part Two — Facilitating Body Confidence.

This book began as an email course. My first test group volunteered to receive email lessons from me five days a week for eight weeks. Some thrived on this daily discipline. Others found this pace too intense to maintain with their already full lives.

The second test group received lessons three days a week for twelve weeks. This worked better for most participants. Consequently, I have written this book with the three-day-a-week format in mind. If you are facilitating this course, I recommend running it as a 12-week course with the first week serving as an introduction to the material and the group and the twelfth week serving as a conclusion to the material and the group.

You may decide to read it all at once to get an overview and then go back and work through the material. Reading the material does not take much time. I have purposely kept the lessons short so they will fit easily into your schedule. However, working through the exercises and integrating the information you gain from them does take time. When working your way through the book, I recommend one chapter per week.

Each chapter is made up of three lessons. Too much material too fast can be overwhelming. On the flip side, if you don't work with the material on a consistent basis, you may be tempted to abandon it.

The danger of going it alone is that life has a way of getting extremely demanding at the same time the material does. If there are things you're not ready, willing, or able to look at or work through, you might decide cleaning the toilets, tackling your taxes, or planning a cross-country move is a better use of your time than finishing the program.

This is why I recommend you join one of my online groups, start a group of your own, or attend one offered by your church, community college, health club, or weight loss center. If you have questions, suggestions, concerns, or success stories, email me at penny@body-confidence.com. I welcome your feedback and would love to hear about your experience. If you'd like individual coaching, this and other information is available at www.body-confidence.com, the Body Confidence website.

If you are facilitating a group, I recommend meeting once a week for 1 or 2 hours. Twelve weeks is the optimal learning time. You should be able to incorporate all three lessons (or one chapter) each week, with the first week serving as an introduction to the course and the twelfth week serving as a closing ceremony. If you can only get an eight-week commitment from participants, you'll need to combine a few chapters.

Whether you are doing this on your own or with a group, there are two key components that are essential to your success. The first is keeping a Body Confidence Journal so you can record your activities, food consumption, goals, insights, emotions, affirmations, and obstacles. At the end of this section, I have included the pages I use in my own Body Confidence Journal. You are welcome to use these or create pages specific to your needs. The journal pages along with worksheets and written exercises for every chapter are available in letter-size format on a CD-ROM, which can be purchased from the publisher.

You don't have to use these pages indefinitely. You do need to use them while you work through this program. In the beginning, it is the best way to become aware of your patterns and chart your progress. If you are short on time or patience, at least use the Daily Recap. It will take you less than two minutes to fill out and will give you an overview of your day. Just by filling out this one form you can gain valuable insight into your attitudes, behaviors, and choices.

If you are working through the program on your own, I recommend using a three-ring binder. Or find a journal that speaks to your creative side, something you will enjoy using and love looking at, touching, and carrying around with you. Without the support of a group, this journal will become the primary witness to your progress. Here you will record your fears, your fantasies, your setbacks, your successes, and the occasional epiphany that changes your life.

If you are facilitating a Body Confidence group, it is imperative that participants get these handouts at the beginning of the course and use them throughout the program. I recommend that facilitators purchase the Body Confidence CD-ROM, which contains letter-size reproducible worksheet masters, and that you provide 3-ring binders for participants to use as their designated Body Confidence Journals. They will be able to store their Daily Recap worksheets along with the weekly handouts and other materials in these binders.

I have included an Awareness Agreement among these worksheets. If you are leading a group, collect these from your participants at the first meeting. If you are doing this on your own, please sign the form on page 163 in this book before beginning. You may also sign the agreement online at www.body-confidence.com. Signing the agreement symbolizes your commitment to yourself and this program.

Throughout this book, I will be encouraging you to incorporate movement and proper nutrition into your lifestyle. I will not be prescribing exercise routines or promoting particular diets. Every "body" is different. Your nutritional needs and training programs will vary depending upon whether you are thirty-something or fifty-something, recovering from an illness or injury, pregnant or nursing a child, trying to lose weight, attempting to gain strength, improve endurance, or increase flexibility. Your job is to discover the way you like to move and the foods that give you the most energy and vitality.

The one thing I will recommend is walking on a regular basis. Unless you have a particular condition or disability that prevents you from walking, there is really no excuse not to walk. It's easy, affordable, and can be done just about anytime or anywhere. I believe there is a "sole to soul" connection that takes place when your feet make contact with the earth. Your body will need to metabolize the information your mind will be digesting. Walking keeps you grounded as your spirit takes flight.

So the second key component to your success is investing in a step counter. Step counters measure the amount of steps you take each day. They serve as excellent motivators to incorporate activity into your schedule. You may be pleasantly surprised to find out how active you already are. Or you may discover you are more sedentary than you suspected. Either way, step counters keep you accountable. I'm addicted to using mine. After three years, it's still a thrill to reach the 10,000 steps per day goal!

Step counters or pedometers range in price from $10 to $40 and measure steps, miles or kilometers, and calories burned — depending on the model. Step counters are small enough to attach to your waistband or pocket. You can find them at sporting goods stores or discount stores. I have listed some sources for step counters in the Introduction section of Resource Central.

If you are facilitating a group, I suggest you contact these companies to secure a discount for your group. If you have any questions about this, email me. Either include the step counters in the price of the course or make them available to your participants at a discount so they do not have to go out and find one on their own. (Don't let the absence of a step counter become an excuse for not using one!)

As a facilitator or group leader, utilize your expertise. If you are a fitness instructor, yoga or meditation teacher/student, therapist, nutritionist, avid walker, etc., incorporate your specialty as part of the group activities. Demonstrating exercises you can do in your chair, practicing belly breathing, showing simple stretches, or leading a pre- or post-workshop walk are excellent additions to the class. A trip to the grocery store to decipher food labels or a cooking class is a fun way to translate the lessons into real life.

What I am providing here is the foundation. What will make your program a success is the enthusiasm, originality, and creativity you bring to it.

If you are not participating in a group, you may decide to work with a personal trainer or nutritionist to supplement this program and expedite your results. As Barbara Sher, author of *Wishcraft* and several other dream building books says, "Isolation is the dream killer." If you don't have a group, then visit the Body Confidence website to receive energetic and electronic support from me.

There are numerous books, videos, and audiotapes devoted to exercise routines, eating plans, and healthy living. I have listed the resources I consulted in the Resource Central section of this book. Explore them! I know what I know because I've had some wonderful teachers. If your favorites are not listed, you are welcome to share your sources of inspiration with others on the Body Confidence website.

Remember to be patient with yourself and the process. It took some time to arrive at the point where you believe you need a course like Body Confidence. It will take some time to reawaken this confidence within you.

Expect to experience glorious days of self-discovery, amazing clarity, and abundant energy. These will usually be followed by horrific days of despair and confusion when you can barely conjure up the energy to get out of bed. On those days you will have to ask yourself what holds more authority over you: your vision for what is possible or your excuses for why it's not.

I am thrilled that you have chosen this path to personal power. Whether you are doing so on your own or in a group, please know I am with you in spirit. Thank you in advance for your courage and commitment.

Daily Recap

Date _____

(Circle the appropriate number. 1=Poor / 5=Excellent)

Activity Level	1	2	3	4	5
Health	1	2	3	4	5
Social Interaction	1	2	3	4	5
Stress Level	1	2	3	4	5
Attitude	1	2	3	4	5

Nutritional Awareness

Breakfast	1	2	3	4	5
Lunch	1	2	3	4	5
Dinner	1	2	3	4	5
Snacks	1	2	3	4	5

Emotional State

Morning	1	2	3	4	5
Afternoon	1	2	3	4	5
Evening	1	2	3	4	5

Overall Daily Totals __ __ __ __ __

Daily Steps (If using Step Counter) _____

NOTES _____
_____
_____
_____
_____

Food Journal

Date _____ Time _____

Amount of food eaten   1   2   3   4   5

Hunger level prior to eating   1   2   3   4   5

Enjoyment of food   1   2   3   4   5

Mood   1   2   3   4   5

Environmental influences _____

_____

_____

Foods eaten _____

_____

_____

_____

Instructions

Time of Day: When did you eat?

Amount: How did you feel when you were finished eating? Rate on a scale of 1 to 5, with 1 being still hungry and 5 being totally stuffed.

Hunger level prior to eating: Rate from 1 to 5, with 1 being not really hungry and 5 being ravenous.

Enjoyment of food: Rate from 1 to 5, with 1 being dislike and 5 being love the taste, texture, smell.

Mood: How were you feeling when you ate? 1 feeling miserable and 5 feeling great.

Environmental influences: What environmental influences added to your desire to eat? The smells? Were other people eating?

Foods eaten: What did you eat?

Workout Journal

Date _____ Time _____

Activity _____

_____

Alone or with someone _____

Time spent on workout _____

Effort exerted/energy level _____

Favorite part _____

Hardest part _____

How I felt before I started _____

How I felt after I finished _____

Any resistance, subtle sabotage _____

Insights, epiphanies, miracles _____

Lower body response _____

Upper body response _____

Properly nourished and hydrated _____

Appropriate breaks and adequate rest _____

Aches or pains / new or old _____

Breakthroughs or goals achieved _____

Best reason to keep at it _____

Notes _____

_____

_____

Goals

Date _____

Goal _____

Why it's worth the effort _____

_____

My plan for reaching this goal _____

_____

Projected date of accomplishment _____

Daily Action Steps

- _____

- _____

- _____

- _____

- _____

Reward _____

Affirmations and inspiration _____

Today's successes/Gratitude list _____

_____

_____

Tomorrow's intentions _____

_____

_____

Chapter One

What Happened?

Lesson 1

Once there was a time when you were mesmerized by the mystery of your body. Your tongue, toes, navel, and nose fascinated you. Each day delivered a sensory smorgasbord of sights, sounds, smells, tastes, and textures for you to explore.

Without even being aware of it, you exuded Body Confidence. Your body was the way you communicated with the world and you never doubted its effectiveness. You could express an entire range of emotions and intentions without a single word.

You were uninhibited. You were eager to show off your body and curious to share your discoveries with others who may have the same or different parts. You were not ashamed of the noises and smells you involuntarily produced. You ate when you were hungry, slept when you were tired, cried when you were cranky, and laughed when you were amused.

And you were probably all of two years old. What power for such a small creature! Then something happened. The balance of power shifted from your body to your brain. Things have not been the same since. Until now.

Now you hold in your hands an invitation to bring your body back into its rightful position of power. Just like the brain, your body's job is to inform your decisions, guide your actions, and keep you healthy. The key is to align your mind and body so you can get the results you intend in all areas of your life.

Staying in your head may have kept you safe and served you well. It probably helped you gloss over your growing dissatisfaction with your body. But if you want to develop Body Confidence, you must be willing to drop down into your body. You must be willing to sweat — to do the physical, mental, emotional, and spiritual work required to move you from your comfort zone to your confidence zone.

Befriending your body is the key to Body Confidence. Treat yourself like you would treat your best friend. Criticizing, name-calling, and verbal abuse contribute to the erosion of Body Confidence. Respect, curiosity, attention, and awareness call it forth.

Putting it into practice

I'd like you to start this process by asking yourself some basic questions: who, what, when, where, why, and how. Before rushing into this interrogation, stop a moment. Take a couple of slow, deep breaths. This will help you center yourself and clear your mind.

Like all the exercises in this book, the answers are primarily for your eyes only. Sharing your answers with someone you trust may be an excellent way for you gain insight into your behavior, and if you are doing this as part of a group, you can learn a great deal from the answers others provide. However, your first responses — the answers that come to you immediately and may or may not make sense — are the most honest and revealing ones. You may be tempted to change or censor them if you fear someone will read and judge your responses. The bottom line is: practice safe sharing.

Who, What, When, Where, Why & How
Exercise 1-1

1. Who do you feel most inhibited or body conscious around?

   _____

   Why? _____

2. Who do you feel least inhibited or body conscious around?

   _____

   Why? _____

3. Who or what shaped your beliefs about your body?

   _____

4. When were you first aware of being ashamed of your body?

   _____

   Where were you? _____

   What were you doing? _____

   Who were you with? _____

   How old were you? _____

5. When were you first aware of being proud of your body?

   _____

   Where were you? _____

   What were you doing? _____

   Who were you with? _____

   How old were you? _____

6. When was the last time you experienced Body Confidence?

   _____

   Where were you?_____

   Who were you with? _____

What were you doing? _____

7. When did you feel your Body Confidence start to diminish?

_____

Why? _____

What event(s) precipitated this decline? _____

_____

8. Who contributed most to the way you perceive yourself?

_____

How did they do this? _____

Does this person continue to influence your perceptions?_____

9. Who did the most damage to your body image? _____

How did they do this? _____

_____

Do they continue to wreak havoc on your relationship with your body?

_____

10. Who do you know who radiates Body Confidence? _____

What do you think is their secret? _____

_____

11. What would you need to do, have, or be to radiate Body Confidence?

_____

What can you do to make this happen? _____

_____

How willing are you to make these adjustments? _____

Why are you willing to commit to this now? _____

_____

Lesson 2

As any good detective knows, once you gather the evidence, you let it speak for itself. Looking over your answers, what does "the evidence" say to you? If you aren't clear, that's okay. This is just the beginning of your stint in internal investigations. Your case will continue to present itself throughout the course of this inquiry. You will see how the stories you have told and tales you continue to tell shape your life.

Once, while Mahatma Gandhi was on a train pulling out of the station, a reporter ran up to him and asked, "Do you have a message I can take back to my people?" Because it was his day of silence, Gandhi did not reply. He simply scrawled on a piece of paper, "My life is my message," and passed it to the reporter.

Guess what? The same is true for you. Your life is your message whether you intend for it to be or not. What are you broadcasting? If you don't know, ask someone — preferably a stranger — if you want unbiased feedback. They can tell you immediately. You may be broadcasting confidence, sophistication, quiet calm, and openness. You may be exuding a sense of depression, fear, anger, or disappointment.

Your posture tends to tell others more about you than your words. And you may not even be aware of it.

In my workshops I do an exercise to illustrate this point. I get out a deck of cards with numbers from 2–10. I ask participants to pick a card and then walk from Point A to Point B "broadcasting" the number on the card. For example, if someone draws a 3, she may walk across the room with her head down, eyes averted, and shoulders slumped. If someone draws a 10, she may look people in the eye, smile, stand tall, and walk purposefully in a specific direction — what I call "walking with power." Other participants receive the broadcast loud and clear. Unfortunately, we forget we are always broadcasting, and that our broadcasts affect how others respond to us.

If the message you are broadcasting is different than you intend, do not despair. You can change channels! However, you must be aware of where you are now.

Putting it into practice

Throughout this book, I will bring you back again and again to the idea of awareness. Before you can initiate any kind of change, you need to be aware of your starting point. For example, if you want to lose weight, you need some kind of measure of how much you weigh right now. You can step on the scales or notice how your clothes fit. When the scales are lighter or your jeans are baggy, then you know you've lost a few pounds. The same concept applies to Body Confidence. In order to develop it, you need to determine your starting point. The following quiz is designed to help you assess your current Body Confidence Quotient.

Body Confidence Quotient (BCQ)
Exercise 1-2

Circle the answers that best describe your behavior.

1. Exercise
    a. I exercise every day.
    b. I exercise 3–4 times a week.
    c. I exercise whenever I can — maybe once a week.
    d. It's on my to-do list — right after I schedule my root canal.

2. Rest
    a. I get plenty of sleep and feel rested and refreshed most days.
    b. I sleep 6–8 hours a night.
    c. I am often sleep deprived.
    d. Who needs to sleep when you have caffeine?

3. Diet
    a. I eat healthy foods and plan most meals around specific dietary guidelines.
    b. I'm conscious of my food choices and eat healthy meals most days.
    c. I do my best given my time, energy, and budget.
    d. I eat whatever I can find between the cushions in my couch.

4. Style
    a. I feel fabulously fashionable in anything I wear. I'm known for starting trends.
    b. I feel fabulous in most of my clothes.
    c. If my clothes fit, that's fabulous.
    d. I'm featured on the Fashion Police "Most Wanted" list.

5. Stress Level
    a. I keep my stress level in check through diet, exercise, meditation, and contemplation.
    b. I manage my responsibilities fairly well and try to stay flexible.
    c. I'm often overwhelmed and underappreciated.
    d. My life is one continuous Stress Fest.

6. Relationships
   a. I'm surrounded by people I love and respect.
   b. I get along well with most of the people in my life.
   c. Many of my relationships are strained.
   d. I don't have the time or energy for relationships.

7. Life Path
   a. I have a clear sense of purpose and seek out situations that support my goals.
   b. I'm happy with the general direction of my life and welcome opportunities to learn.
   c. I don't know what path I'm on, but I'm getting there as quickly as I can.
   d. My mission is to get through the day.

8. Environment
   a. My surroundings support my health and well-being on all levels.
   b. My surroundings are clean, comfortable, and life enhancing.
   c. My surroundings are sufficient.
   d. Are there any feng shui cures for a cardboard box?

9. Energy Level
   a. I have energy to burn and can easily meet the demands of my full life.
   b. I have enough energy to manage most days.
   c. I can get through the day if I have an ample supply of chocolate and caffeine.
   d. I only have enough energy to change my mind.

10. Charisma
   a. I light up a room when I walk in.
   b. I am comfortable in new situations and enjoy meeting new people.
   c. I feel uncomfortable in new situations and prefer being with people I know.
   d. I light up a room when I walk out.

BONUS QUESTION: Ms. America Contest
  a. I would win based on the swimsuit competition.
  b. I would win based on the evening gown competition.
  c. I would win based on the talent competition.
  d. I would win based on my ideas for bringing about world peace.

Your Body Confidence Quotient

If you circled mostly a's — Honey, you can cheer the rest of us on because you have Body Confidence to boot. I assume you are reading this book to make sure I have included everything you already possess. You are an inspiration. Rock on.

If you circled mostly b's — Perfection is overrated, yes? You have mastered the art of living well and are to be commended. I assume you are reading this book because you are continually looking for ways to improve yourself. You have heard these ideas before. Maybe now, grasshopper, you will consistently put them into practice.

If you circled mostly c's — Help is on the way! You have a demanding life and are doing your best to keep your head above water. I assume you are reading this book because it represents a lifeboat thrown from the mother-ship. Here's my challenge to you, lotus blossom. Would you be willing to float until the boat can reach you? It takes far less effort and is actually rejuvenating. Of course, you must believe the very water that threatens to drown you will also support you. Can you stop struggling long enough to see the lifeboat sailing in your direction?

If you circled mostly d's — Your core of confidence has been crushed. Fortunately, your sense of humor remains intact.

Lesson 3

You now have a sense of where you are on the Body Confidence continuum. You have started your investigation into the people, places, and events that caused your confidence to erode or emerge. You have discovered that what you say, how you move, and the way you act broadcast a message about your life.

As you may have guessed, I included 4's simply for comic relief. Even though developing Body Confidence is a serious pursuit, it's vital that you not take yourself too seriously. There is fun to be had along the way! And I want you to have some.

Putting it into practice

So the last exercise for the week is to have some fun. I'd like you to write down 15 things you love to do. You don't have to do these things often or do them well, but you must love to do them. Because if you truly love them, you'll get energized just thinking about them.

Once you have your list in front of you, check off the things you have done in the last week, the last month, or the last year. Does feeling good in the skin you're in affect your enjoyment of the activity? Is there something on your list you would be willing to treat yourself to today?

Body Confidence starts right now. Whether you complete this program in twelve days, twelve weeks, or twelve months, the benefits start the moment you decide Body Confidence is your birthright and claim your right to it.

Fifteen Things I Love To Do

Exercise 1-3

Write down 15 things you love to do. Then check off when you last did them.

Activity	This Week	This Month	This Year
1.			
2.			
3.			
4.			
5.			
6.			
7.			
8.			
9.			
10.			
11.			
12.			
13.			
14.			
15.			

Chapter Two

Start Where You Are

Lesson 4

To begin a program such as Body Confidence takes a significant amount of courage because what you are doing is inviting change into your life. Although you might make the assumption that changing specific things about your life — like losing weight or gaining strength — will bring about previously unbeknownst bliss, the reality of initiating such a change is still daunting. Desired changes are often accompanied by random and unruly changes.

There is a seductive sense of security in knowing that happiness is only ten pounds away. There is a distorted sense of power in this delayed gratification of sorts. In her book, *Making Peace with Food*, Susan Kano calls this "delusions of slender grandeur." If you believe you will be able to do any number of things you can't do now if you were only 10–20–30 pounds lighter, you're suffering from this syndrome.

Change happens whether you initiate it or not. Your body tends to register this fact more quickly than your mind. Whether you take up kickboxing, stop eating meat, drink green tea, practice yoga, or run with the wolves, your body knows that what you can do today is different from what you could do yesterday.

This may mean your body functions better than ever. Or it may mean the awe and delight you felt for your body at one point has been replaced by disbelief, suspicion, disappointment, and even disgust. Instead of working with your body and giving it what it needs, you've declared war on your buns, belly, breasts, and biceps. You've withheld food and other essentials from it in order to force it to comply with your demands.

As a fitness instructor for almost two decades, my heart aches at the collective anguish people suffer in relationship to their bodies. They dutifully diet, endlessly exercise, and wearily weigh in despite their deepest fear that all this suffering might be for nothing.

The good news is the suffering can be over. The not-so-good news is you have to surrender. You have to give up your attachments to images of the ideal or pictures of perfection portrayed by movies, magazines, and models. And even if you let go of these images, they will continue to permeate our culture and influence others' behavior. Since this falls into the "beyond your control" category, it is not your concern at this point.

Your focus during this course will be on what is within your control. I call these your ABC's — attitudes, behaviors, and choices. We'll start by uncovering what they are.

Putting it into practice

Your first workout is a speed-writing exercise. What speed-writing does is capture your first (and usually truest) response. The first page is a list of questions regarding your beliefs about your body. The second page is an answer sheet.

The best way to complete this exercise is to have someone you trust read the questions to you. Take a moment to get centered. Taking a few deep breaths may do the trick. Once the question is read, respond within 5–10 seconds max. The goal is to answer the questions as quickly as possible with the first response that comes to mind. You can read the questions yourself and fill in the answers, but this tempts you to spend too much time answering the question.

Speed Writing Questions
Exercise 2-1

1. My favorite activity is ...

2. The last meal I truly enjoyed was ...

3. The thing I really love about my body is ...

4. The thing I feel most ashamed or embarrassed about is ...

5. When I was a child the message I got about my body was ...

6. I get the most energy from ...

7. The types of foods I like to eat are generally ...

8. I was most proud of the way I looked when I was ...

9. If I were an elite athlete, I'd be ...

10. I carry stress in this part of my body ...

11. If I could change one thing about my appearance it would be ...

12. I'm often complimented on my ...

13. If my body had one message for me right now it would be ...

14. I remember being very sick when ...

15. Of all my senses, I rely most heavily on my sense of ...

On a scale of 1-10 with 1 mostly true and 10 mostly false, rate the following:

16. Appearance is important to my family and friends.

17. I am comfortable with my sexuality.

18. I believe illness is a sign of weakness.

19. I accept myself for being less than perfect.

20. I savor sensual pleasures like massages, walking barefoot in the sand, or soaking in the tub.

Speed Writing Answers
Exercise 2-1

1. _____
2. _____
3. _____
4. _____
5. _____
6. _____
7. _____
8. _____
9. _____
10. _____
11. _____
12. _____
13. _____
14. _____
15. _____
16.   1   2   3   4   5   6   7   8   9   10
17.   1   2   3   4   5   6   7   8   9   10
18.   1   2   3   4   5   6   7   8   9   10
19.   1   2   3   4   5   6   7   8   9   10
20.   1   2   3   4   5   6   7   8   9   10

Lesson 5

Were you surprised by your answers to the speed writing assignment? It's a good idea to re-examine your beliefs on a regular basis. Whether you realize it or not, beliefs you formed about yourself and your body at age 5, 16, or 21 may still be influencing the way you perceive yourself now.

What stories are you carrying around about yourself that may or may not be true? What life events have limited you from becoming stronger, more flexible, or more active in general? What events have inspired you to break through your limits?

I'm going to spend a lot of time in this course helping you get current. In other words, I want to help you figure out what patterns formed in the past are preventing you from being all you are capable of being right now. Then we'll figure out what actions you can take today that will shape your future.

To create a different future you must first be able to imagine it. Fast forward 3–6–12 months down the road. If everything goes as planned and you are quite confident in your own skin, what will be different? What will you be doing? What will you be eating? How will you be feeling? Who will you have around you? What actions, behaviors, and choices will have shifted in order to make this transformation possible? Your answers will serve as your blueprint and guide today's actions.

Putting it into practice

Here's what I'd like you to do. First, put on your walking shoes. The best way to link up your mind and body is to get moving. Refuse to listen to the voices reminding you of the hundreds of other things you need to do besides walk. Trust me, alphabetizing the canned goods can wait for thirty minutes. (Yes, these voices are not only ridiculous, but also relentless!)

Give yourself a good 20–30 minutes to walk down memory lane and dig up some vital information. Whether you choose to walk on a tread-mill or hit the hiking trail, try to find a place relatively free of distractions so you can turn your focus inward.

Since I'm not there with you, I'm depending on you to determine the amount of time and level of intensity that is appropriate for you. As a rule of thumb, you should be able to carry on a conversation with someone while you walk. (Of course today, you'll be talking to yourself.) If you're too winded to string at least five words together, you're working at a pretty intense level and may want to slow down a bit.

Once you get moving, think back on your life and identify three or four significant events that formed your identity as either "an athlete" or "a spectator." What or who made you believe that anything you demanded from your body was either possible or impossible? How old were you? Who else was involved? What was happening in your life at the time? How have these events influenced your image of yourself today? You can use the worksheet that follows to record your answers.

For example, when I was 20, I was an exchange student at McGill University in Montreal, Canada. I was there to study French, but my unspoken desire was to dance. I joined a dance class, and one day the instructor came up to me and asked me what I was doing in Montreal. I told her I was studying French. Then she said the words that validated my private passion. "You should be studying dance." I danced on air for months after that.

Although I didn't drop out of college to pursue a dancing career, I eventually became a fitness professional and an "aerobic dancer." This reinforced my perception of myself as an athlete. As an athlete, I attempt things (like a seated butt drop on my nieces' trampoline) that I might not try if I considered myself a spectator.

End your walk with some gentle stretches. Then before you head for the canned goods, notice what it feels like to be in your body. If you're like most people, you spend more time in your head than your body. Take a moment to drop down into your body and just listen. You might just be amazed at what you hear!

Do you feel refreshed by a slight chill in the air that adds color to your cheeks? Do you feel like you've pushed through mental blocks as well as physical ones when you finally break a sweat? Do your legs feel energized? How does your upper body feel when it's in motion?

Before the exercise high wears off, capture your experience in your journal. You can use Today's Workout from your BC Journal pages to answer the exercise awareness questions. You can use the following pages for the Athlete or Spectator exercise. Or you may want to write about something else that struck you as significant while you were walking. Even if it seems totally unrelated to my questions, jot it down. You never know where a kernel of truth will take you.

Enjoy your walk!

Athlete or Spectator
Exercise 2-2

Think back on your life and identify three or four significant events that formed your identity as either "an athlete" or "a spectator." Consider the following questions:

• Did this event make you believe anything you demanded from your body was possible or impossible?

• How old were you?

• Who else was involved?

• What was happening in your life at the time?

• How have these events influenced your image of yourself today?

Significant Event: _____

Age: _____ Athlete or Spectator: _____

Impact: _____

_____

Significant Event: _____

Age: _____ Athlete or Spectator: _____

Impact: _____

_____

Significant Event: _____

Age: _____ Athlete or Spectator: _____

Impact: _____

_____

Significant Event: _____

Age: _____ Athlete or Spectator: _____

Impact: _____

_____

Lesson 6

How was the walk? Did any significant stories surface that shed some light on your relationship with your body? Did you have mostly empowering or disempowering stories?

Today's lesson may be the toughest one all week. I want you to fall in love. I'm sure you have experienced the magic of falling in love — whether it was with your mate, your child, your pet, or your favorite place.

Do you remember how everything looks brighter through the lens of love? Everything about the beloved is fascinating. Your senses are stimulated in ways you previously overlooked. You are free with your forgiveness. You are generous with your joy. You give yourself permission to temporarily suspend judgment.

That's exactly what I'd like you to do for yourself throughout this course. Temporarily suspend judgment. Just observe. Notice. Pay attention. Make choices. Make different choices. There will be no self-loathing while you're in my company.

I want you to begin to grasp how amazing you are. I want you to focus not on what's wrong with you but on what's right with you. I would like you not to worry about what you look like to others but how you appear to yourself. I hope to banish your fears of growing old or getting ill by introducing you to your own personal power supply.

You see, Body Confidence begins right now — not in eight weeks or six months or a year from now when you feel fabulous and look marvelous. Body Confidence is an attitude you develop every day by choosing beliefs and actions that support your inner vision.

Putting it into practice

This weekend I encourage you to get out and get moving. Do something you love to do, even if you haven't done it in years. If nothing comes to mind, refer back to your 15 Things I Love To Do list, pick one, and do it.

Got an old hula hoop in your garage? Get it out and swivel those hips! How about a bike ride or game of golf? What about an impromptu dance around the kitchen with your partner, kids, or a good broom?

After you get those endorphins flowing, take a few moments and fill out the Progress Report on the following page. Throughout the program, I'd like you to check your motivation level. As I mentioned in the Introduction, it's not that you don't know how to lose weight or eat right or gain strength. More often it's that you don't know how to stay motivated to reach your goals.

The Progress Report is similar to the Daily Recap, except it asks you to summarize your cumulative progress. It gives you a big picture perspective (what Jamie Sams, in her books on Native American wisdom, calls "eagle vision") as opposed to the daily details ("mouse vision"). Both perspectives are necessary to keep you on track, but using your eagle vision allows you to spot trends or patterns that you may overlook using mouse vision.

Progress Report
Exercise 2-3

Date _____

	(1=Poor / 5=Excellent)				
Activity Level	1	2	3	4	5
Health	1	2	3	4	5
Social Interaction	1	2	3	4	5
Stress Level	1	2	3	4	5
Attitude	1	2	3	4	5
Nutritional Awareness	1	2	3	4	5
Emotional State	1	2	3	4	5
Overall	1	2	3	4	5

What have I enjoyed the most about this program? What have I discovered about myself, my body, my likes and dislikes?

_____

_____

_____

What is the most challenging part of this program? What situations or
circumstances cause me to question my resolve or intentions?

_____

_____

_____

What reinforcement do I need — more information, a support group,
exercise equipment, more fruits and vegetables in the house?

_____

_____

_____

What patterns are emerging regarding my activity level?

_____

_____

_____

What patterns are emerging regarding my nutritional awareness?

_____

_____

_____

What patterns are emerging regarding my attitudes or emotional state?

_____

_____

_____

What patterns are emerging regarding my social interactions?

_____

_____

_____

What do I need to do more of to stay motivated and on track?

_____

_____

_____

What do I need to do less of to stay motivated and on track?

_____

_____

_____

Chapter Three

Examine Your Expectations

Lesson Seven

When it comes to reaching your goal, expectations can play a significant part in your success or failure. Unexamined expectations are often the culprits that cause you to quit your program just when you're starting to gain momentum.

Let's start by examining the expectations you may have of others. You will need a good deal of courage and commitment to make changes in your lifestyle. You will also need to solicit the support of those around you.

It's easy to underestimate the effect your changes have on those close to you. Some people may be downright threatened by your decision to become a vegetarian, join a spinning class, or go on a silent retreat. Forget the fact that it's in your best interest to do so. If it's not necessarily in theirs, they (whoever they may be) are not going to make it easy for you.

It's not because they don't love you. Ironically, they may be the very people who love you the most. And they love you "just the way you are." So when you decide to change the way you are, things can get a little complicated.

When you pass up the pizza party and movie marathon in favor of a walk in the park, prepare to have your new lifestyle and choices criticized. Your actions might move your friends and family out of their comfort zone. Of course, this may be a good thing! They just might not see it that way.

As you consider the changes you'd like to make, also consider how these changes will impact your friends, family, and community. Hopefully, you will be an inspiration to all you meet! Realistically, your results may not elicit your desired response.

This is where we can support each other. Resolutions that meet with too much resistance and not enough reinforcement eventually fail. Expect resistance to this program — both internal and external. When you understand where the resistance comes from and why, you will be able to work with it.

Putting it into practice

If you can't find 20–30 minutes to walk, snatch 5–10 minutes every hour (or two at the most) to walk down the hall, climb the stairs, or stretch out your muscles. At each of these intervals, pick one of the questions from the following worksheet as the focus of your "mini-workout." When you return to your desk, drink a glass of water. Then jot down a quick answer to the question you picked.

Support System
Exercise 3-1

1. Who might benefit the most from the changes I want to make?

   _____

2. Who might benefit the least from the changes I want to make?

   _____

3. How will the changes affect my relationships with my family, friends, or community?

   _____

   _____

4. How many of my current activities revolve around food?

   _____

5. How many of my current activities revolve around fitness?

   _____

6. Do most of my family and friends make healthy choices? _____

7. Does my work environment promote healthy living? _____

8. How accessible is a fitness facility or workout studio?

   _____

9. Do my friends and family lead an active lifestyle?

   _____

10. Who might support me and who might resist me in my effort to lose weight, get fit, etc.?

    Support: _____

    Resist: _____

Lesson 8

What did you learn about your current support system? Is it one that will welcome the changes you seek to make or subtly sabotage them? What do you need to do to gain support from those who are important to you?

It's the little things that can make or break your resolve. My goal for our work together is to help you identify and overcome these obstacles.

As I mentioned in the introduction, there are many excellent books, programs, and videos that will give you the specifics of what to eat and why as well as when to exercise and how. You can decide what program or guidelines you want to follow for your external fitness program.

In this course, I am concerned with the internal obstacles that keep you from feeling fabulous. These obstacles — many of them unrealistic expectations — mess with your success and rob you of the joy of being in your body.

Of course, not all expectations are unrealistic. In fact, you need realistic expectations in order to accomplish your goal. For example: "I expect to exercise three times a week for 30 minutes and pay attention to my portion sizes at meals." "I expect to be patient and am happy to lose 1–2 pounds a week." "I expect to stay motivated during this course." "I expect to experience some resistance as I make changes in my lifestyle."

Realistic expectations are the ones you readily admit to. It's the ones you don't admit to that I'm concerned about. Those are the ones that are running the show and ultimately responsible if you abandon your agenda. For example, "I expect to see significant improvement, but I will only exercise when I feel like it, eat what I want, and write in my journal when I have time."

Naturally these expectations are not going to present themselves in such an obvious manner. They usually surface more subtly, such as when a coworker brings a birthday cake to the office the day you decide to cut down on sweets. Or a friend invites you to dinner the same night as your yoga class. Or a family member phones to chat during the 20 minutes you've managed to sequester for yourself to reflect and write in your journal.

Do not interpret these events as the universe conspiring to keep you out of shape, overweight, or overwhelmed. Instead, try to see each event as an opportunity to make a choice that either supports your new goals or reinforces your old habits.

Forget feeling guilty. Just notice the circumstances that allow you to make positive choices and the circumstance that lead you make poor ones. Awareness is the key to creating any kind of change.

As you go through this course, keep your expectations in check. Try not to let your expectations of what should be happening overshadow what is happening.

Putting it into practice

What is the most enjoyable way you can put yourself in motion today? How about a swim, a stretch class, a tennis match, or an afternoon of serious gardening? Decide what will get your heart pumping and singing. Commit to carrying it out today.

After you've moved around and settled into your body, take a few minutes to notice some of the expectations you have about your body. The important word here is notice — not judge, criticize, or comment. Regardless of how outrageous they may seem once you identify them, record your expectations on the following page.

Here are a few of my more "interesting" expectations regarding my body.

- I expect my body to perform at optimal levels even when I feed it junk food and don't exercise.

- I expect to be healthy and feel great all the time.

- I expect to lose weight without doing anything differently.

- I expect exercise to be easy and effortless.

- I expect to look like the people in the exercise videos even though I'm eating ice cream as I "preview" them.

- I expect someone else to prepare delicious and nutritious meals for me.

- I expect to be in great shape without having to work at it.

- I expect to be younger, richer, and sexier when I'm 15 pounds lighter.

- I expect to feel full of energy every morning regardless of what I did or consumed the night before.

Okay, your turn. Don't hold back.

Expectations
Exercise 3-2

Write down any and all expectations you have of yourself and this program. After you have written them down, look them over and put a check next to any expectations that might seem a bit unrealistic and could sabotage your progress.

I expect _____

_____

I expect _____

_____

I expect _____

_____

I expect _____

_____

I expect _____

_____

I expect _____

_____

I expect _____

_____

I expect _____

_____

I expect _____

_____

I expect _____

_____

Lesson 9

Sometimes you inherit your expectations. Like heavy hips, broad shoulders, or poor coordination, you might assume that if your parents, gender, or nationality struggles with certain tendencies, you must too.

There's no denying DNA. But there are options available to deal with your genetic predispositions. If you are prone to particular physical characteristics, such as an ample abdomen or generous gluteus maximus, you can learn how eating the right foods and doing certain exercises can help you work with what you've got.

If you're predisposed toward certain illnesses like diabetes or heart disease, eating right and exercising will go a long way toward preserving your health as well. As Caroline Myss says, when "our biology becomes our biography," we often forget we have the option of rewriting the script.

Whether you realize it or not, you have a running story about your health. You may not have articulated it to anyone, but it still influences your actions. For example, if you sprained your right ankle several times, you may avoid doing certain things because you believe you have a weak right ankle. If your mother, grandmother, and great-grandmother suffered a heart attack before they reached 60, you may assume you are going to suffer a similar fate.

If these stories inspire you to take preventive measures, they serve you well. If they limit you to a fate that leaves you feeling powerless, it's time to rewrite the story.

Putting it into practice

This weekend recruit your kids, spouse, friends, neighbors, or pets to accompany you on a walk through the park, a bike ride around the block, or a day on the ski slopes. After all, you're not the only one who can benefit from exercising or spending time in nature.

Of course, if they pass up this opportunity of the week, that doesn't mean you should too. As Gandhi said, "Be the change you seek in the world." Set the example. Do the right thing. Get yourself in motion.

Find ways to move that are fun for you. Your body is designed for movement and pleasure. If you've forgotten the bliss of being in your body, visit a playground and take notes from the kids.

Sometime over the weekend consider the following questions about your family of origin and the environment in which you grew up. Then answer the same questions about your current family environment. If you live alone, answer the questions with regard to your friends and community.

Family of Origin
Exercise 3-3

1. What did your family look like? (physical characteristics)

   _____

2. Did your relatives tend to be large or small people? _____

3. Were they active or sedentary? _____

4. Were family members healthy or ill? _____

5. What kind of foods did you eat? _____

   _____

6. How did your house smell? _____

7. Were meal times happy gatherings or fearful and unpredictable

   confrontations? _____

8. How did you celebrate special events? _____

   _____

9. What kinds of food were considered special treats? _____

   _____

10. Who did the shopping, the cooking, the cleaning up? _____

    _____

11. Did you go out for meals often? _____

12. Did social gatherings revolve around food or activities? _____

13. What kind of energy filled the house? _____

14. Was there lots laughter in your home or mainly silence?

    _____

15. What did you love to do? _____

    _____

Current Family or Community
Exercise 3-3

1. What does your family look like now? _____

_____

2. Is your family active or sedentary? _____

3. Are your family members healthy or ill? _____

4. What kind of foods do you eat? _____

_____

5. How does your house smell? _____

6. Are meal times happy gatherings or fearful and unpredictable

confrontations? _____

7. How do you celebrate special events? _____

_____

8. What foods do you consider special treats? _____

_____

9. Who does the shopping, the cooking, the cleaning up? _____

_____

10. Do you go out for meals often? _____

11. Do your social gatherings revolve around food or activities?

_____

12. What kind of energy fills your house? _____

13. Is there lots laughter in your home or mainly silence?

_____

14. What do you love to do? _____

_____

Chapter Four

Explore Your Options

Lesson 10

It's easy to be overwhelmed by the seemingly endless choices involved in determining the appropriate exercise program, shopping for nutritious food, or following a weight loss program. Part of your journey is to discover what works for you and what doesn't. Yes, it would be nice if there were a simple solution. But you are a complex creature who is different today than you were yesterday. Your body requires different things from you at different ages, different activity levels, and in different environments. Once you tune in to your body you'll be able to register these changes as they occur.

One thing that remains relatively stable is your personality style. Knowing your basic preferences can cut down on some of the options available to you, making your choices clearer and less overwhelming. I've included an eating and exercise profile that may help you determine the strengths and challenges inherent in your preferred style.

Once you determine your personality profile, record it in your journal. This will help you determine what you need to succeed. You may want to make of note of these things as well. For example, what do you need from a workout? What do you need from an eating plan? How can you meet these needs?

If you haven't implemented the use of the Daily Recap forms I provided at the beginning of the book, I urge you to start using them now. Even if it isn't your preferred style to write things down, the best way to become aware of your habits, patterns, and overall preferences is to keep a record of them.

You may also want to record what's going on in your life in general. Have you been having strange dreams lately? Write them down. Is a certain song running through your head? Jot down the lyrics and see if there is a message for you. Did a book fall off the shelf when you walked by? Notice the title or open it up to a random page and see what it has to say.

As you drop down into your body, messages will emerge. Listen. Your body is always attempting to offer up its wisdom. Are you willing to listen?

Putting it into practice

We all have preferences when it comes to dieting and exercise. Read over the descriptions and see which ones apply to you. You may be a combination of all three. Identifying your dominant personality preferences can help you make appropriate choices. Choose the number that most closely resembles your preferences.

What's Your Preference?
Exercise 4-1

Circle the number that best represents your style.

Eating Plans

1 I need details and plans. I like to be told when, what, and how much to eat. I prefer structure. Having too many choices leads to temptation and frustration.

2 I like having specific guidelines so I know how it's "supposed" to be done, but I don't always follow them. I use the ideas but depend on my own creativity to make a plan that works for me.

3 "I don't make the rules. I just break them." I need freedom and lots of choices. I do better when I listen to my gut.

Tracking Progress

1 I rely on the scales. Numbers don't lie.

2 I'll weigh myself but consider the big picture. My average weight loss shows me how well I'm progressing.

3 What scale? If my clothes are too tight, my plan is not working. If my clothes are getting loose, my plan is working.

Cooking/Shopping

1 If it worked for me before, it will work again. I stick to a plan. No use reinventing the wheel. I don't leave home without a list.

2 I'll use what's worked before, but I like to find new ways to prepare my meals. I'll make a list but feel free substitute similar items that are more appealing.

3 That was then. This is now. I'll need to find new and exciting ways to prepare my meals. What's in season? What mood am I in? What color will round out my aesthetic experience?

Exercising

1 I like to work with a trainer so I know what to do. I like having my workouts supervised and my progress charted.

2 I like to take classes so I can learn new things and stay motivated. Attending classes helps me chart my activity level; plus it gives me the option of exercising the way I enjoy most.

3 Give me wide-open spaces and exercise shoes. I prefer to create my own adventures and take on whatever challenges arise.

Interpreting the Results

If your answers are mostly 1s, your style is Dependably Detailed.
Your strengths:

- You're likely to keep a journal of your progress.
- You're likely to see regular weight loss and fitness gains.
- You're likely to feel in control of your diet and exercise plan.

What you need to be aware of:

- You may be more likely to quit than to change the rules or live up to your own expectations.
- You may deprive yourself of forbidden food or pleasures and then feel guilty if you indulge.
- You may get bored with doing the same activities and eating the same foods all the time.
- "All or nothing" thinking may prove too stressful.

If your answers are mostly 2s, your style is Creatively Conscious.
Your strengths:

- You're likely to adapt well to the changes inherent in behavior modification programs.
- You're likely to keep track of what's working and what's not working and make adjustments.
- You're likely to use several strategies to reach your goals.

What you need to be aware of:

- You may allow yourself too much flexibility and get distracted.
- You may be inconsistent in your efforts to reach your goal.
- You may get careless over time and not be accountable enough in one or two areas to reach your overall goal.

If your answers are mostly 3s, your style is Ferociously Free.
Your strengths:

- You're likely to try new food and activities so you won't get bored.
- You're likely to make the changes fit your lifestyle.
- You're likely to reward yourself often which helps you stay motivated.

What you need to be aware of:

- Your choices may be overwhelming, making smart choices difficult to decipher.
- You may not know how to get where you want to go without a "map" or any guidelines.
- You're less likely to plan ahead and be prepared for situational sabotage.
- You're less likely to keep track of your progress or write in your journal.

Lesson 11

Did it help to identify your diet and exercising personality? Sometimes, pointing out the obvious can trigger an epiphany. Now that you know the strengths and possible pitfalls of your personality preference, you will be able to negotiate your choices with greater awareness.

Cheri Huber of the Zen Mountain Center has written a book called *How You Do Anything Is How You Do Everything: A Workbook*. I've come to appreciate the truth of this title each time I attempt a new set of skills or a behavior change.

Many of the issues I have with money are similar to the ones I have with food. Some of the issues I have with relationships are similar to the ones I have with my body. It's not possible to make decisions about one area of my life without it impacting the rest of my life. It comes down to the sum total of who I am being greater than the individual parts.

Just for kicks, I'd like you to draw some unlikely conclusions about your experiences. What parts of your life might be operating under a similar set of assumptions? How might losing weight impact your bottom line financially? How could being present and paying attention to how you prepare your food influence how you relate to others? How might starting a strength-training program prompt a career move?

I'm a firm believer that as you become more flexible in your body, you will become more flexible in other areas of your life. As you become stronger in your body, you will become stronger and more committed to your vision and values. As you become more aerobically fit, you will be able to practice patience and realize long-term goals.

By adding stretching, strength training, and aerobic work to your routine, you not only transform your body but your soul. After years of putting up with an unappreciative boss, you might find the courage to state your needs or change positions. After resisting certain procedures or policies, you might find yourself able to bend a little in your position. You might even be able to tolerate the wait at the Department of Motor Vehicles by repeating a mantra or practicing a little office yoga. Anything is possible!

Putting it into practice

Notice the interconnectedness of things. My favorite way to do this is to put on my walking shoes and head outside. I always find at least one treasure when I'm out walking. I've collected innumerable rocks, shells, feathers — even a few dogs have followed me home — but that's another story.

Pick up one such treasure (maybe a stone or a feather) and then create a story about how it came to be on your path on this day. You are now the caretaker of this treasure. What is your history together? What is your future? How will this treasure assist you on your journey toward health and well-being?

Let this treasure become your talisman throughout your journey. Whenever you feel like giving up, draw on it for strength. Whenever you feel you are not enough, let it remind you of how much more you are. You need reminders of your beauty. Let this treasure be your reminder.

Treasure Hunt
Exercise 4-2

1. What did you find? _____

   _____

2. How did it come upon your path on this day? _____

   _____

3. What is its story? _____

   _____

   _____

   _____

4. What drew you to it? _____

   _____

5. How does it radiate the qualities you need on your path?_____

   _____

6. What can you do to honor it? _____

   _____

7. What can you do to honor yourself? _____

   _____

8. What is it helping you find?_____

   _____

9. Does it have a sacred name or place? _____

   _____

10. How do you feel as its caretaker? _____

    _____

    _____

Lesson 12

As I mentioned in the Introduction, fitness and weight-loss programs generally don't fail because you don't know how to lose weight or gain strength, increase flexibility or endurance. They fail because you don't know how to stay motivated to maintain these new habits.

"Practice, practice, practice" can lose its appeal after awhile.

Let's consider for a moment how many habits you unconsciously re-inforce day in and day out. How many things are you doing, saying, or thinking without connecting to the truth of that action, statement, or thought?

How often do you find yourself saying things like, "I'd love to exercise, but I'm too busy right now?" "I'd love to buy more nutritious foods, but I can't afford them." "I'd love to learn to meditate, but I'm too stressed to slow down."

If I asked you to meet me for a walk this evening, what would your first response be: "I'd love to!" or "I'd love to, but . . . "?

There's no right or wrong answer. Just notice what comes up for you. Does your body instinctively open up or shut down?

Like having a baby, building a house, planning a career move, or chart-ing a family vacation, timing is everything. Certain elements need to be in place before you can comfortably commit to changes of this caliber.

However, as many of you may know, nothing can prepare you for par-enthood like being a parent. Nothing will prepare you for the infinite decisions involved in building a house except building it. Researching a company's financial future will not tell you whether you'll be a wel-come addition to their baseball team. Watching the weather channel for a month before your vacation cannot predict the freak tornado you may encounter on your bike riding tour of Italy.

At some point you have to take a leap of faith. You have to trust yourself enough to know that whatever comes up, you can handle it. You have to trust yourself enough to know that given any number of choices, you will make the "right" one. And if you don't, you can choose again. And again!

Throughout this book I'll share some ideas about what "right" choices might look like if your goal is eating more nutritious foods, losing weight, gaining strength, increasing your flexibility, or increasing your endurance. But to make this work for you, you can't just take my word for it.

You're going to have to bring a conscious awareness to your activities — shopping, cooking, eating, exercising, resting, etc. Hopefully you already have. If so, keep it up! If not, this is the time to commit to it.

Putting it into practice

The sheer number of decisions required to order a sandwich at a local sub shop can lead to an overwhelmed woman's undoing. While major decisions are often made without difficulty, the deluge of daily decisions can paralyze the practicing perfectionist.

To keep analysis paralysis in check, consider making choices more fun by eliminating the "wrong decision" verdict. Why not consider your choices "intriguing," "fascinating," "revealing," or "inspired"?

Sometimes the paralysis springs from believing you have no choice. But just remember YAHOO — You Always Have Other Options. (Yes, that's where the search engine name originated.)

Here are a few opportunities to explore your options.

The Choice Is Yours
Exercise 4-3

1. What color is your favorite food? _____

2. What time of day do you have the most energy?

   _____

3. How much sleep do you need? _____

4. How does your body feel when deprived of sleep?_____

   _____

5. Who or what gives you energy? _____

6. What physical sensations do you experience when you are energized?

   _____

7. Who or what drains your energy? _____

8. What physical sensations do you experience when you are feeling drained?

   _____

9. What climate do you prefer to exercise in — "controlled" indoor or "anything goes" outdoor?

   _____

10. Do you like to exercise alone or with someone? _____

11. Do you like a regular routine or need spontaneous adventures?

    _____

12. How often do these answers change?

    _____

GOAL: See if you can discover something new or debunk some of the myths you've been perpetuating about yourself.

Chapter Five

Lighten Your Load

Lesson 13

There are very few people I know — women in particular — who wouldn't prefer to be 10–20 pounds lighter rather than 10–20 pounds heavier. Even if the method of losing this weight might jeopardize their health, many people are willing to pay the price.

On any given day, almost half of all American women are on a diet. Thirty-six million people head to health clubs to help them achieve their fitness goals. Eight million people last year sought out a surgical solution.

While images of youth, athleticism, and airbrushed beauty are constantly presented by the media as the ideal, the real deal is that most people are not comfortable in their own skin. Many people feel disconnected from their own source of power and rely on food to fill this emptiness. Consequently, three times as many people in this country have an eating disorder than have AIDS.

Because I came close to losing my life to anorexia as a teenager, I have plenty to say about this subject. I won't pretend to do it justice in one chapter. However, no talk about Body Confidence can be complete without acknowledging "the dark side."

In our exuberance to achieve our goals, our best intentions can turn into obsessive or compulsive behaviors that ultimately lead to self destruction. If you have a healthy sense of self to start with, this may not be an issue. But I'm guessing you are reading this because your Body Confidence needs a boost. If you are considering taking a short cut that compromises your health, please reconsider. "Dying to be thin" is too high a price for you to pay.

After all, the focus of Body Confidence is not losing weight but gaining confidence in your ability to create and maintain a healthy body. It's about accepting and loving who you are regardless of the number on the scales. While you may agree with this idea in principle, the moment you step on the scales another — more emotionally driven — reality takes over.

In her book, *The Dance*, Oriah Mountain Dreamer poses the question, "What if the question is not why am I so infrequently the person I really want to be, but why do I so infrequently want to be the person I really am?" She goes on to explore the obsession with thinking we must be smarter, sexier, thinner, and more stylish to be acceptable.

What if you could accept that who you are is enough? Of course your body complains when you begin to exercise in earnest. Naturally your mind revolts at the thought of abstaining from chocolate. It's possible the fashion police will fine you if you wear your favorite t-shirt to a formal event. But isn't this what makes you fascinating?

I'm not suggesting you give up your goals or deny your innate desire to evolve. I am suggesting that once you come to terms with who you are and give up the idea that you are not enough, perhaps you will finally see that you are.

If you are tormenting yourself about your weight, would you be willing to stop doing so long enough for me to suggest your value as a person cannot be measured in pounds? Before you assure me you'd never equate your weight with your worth, consider the times you have.

Putting it into practice

Do you ever look in the mirror and start slinging any number of insults at yourself, all revolving around some variation of the "I'm too fat" theme? Did you ever stop to ask yourself what you're "too fat" for? Are you too fat to organize an event? Are you too fat to have children or grandchildren? Are you too fat to sing? Are you too fat to enjoy a sunset? Are you too fat to be loved? How fat is "too fat" and who determines that? Do you discriminate against fat people? What assumptions do you make about them? Let's find out.

On the Fat vs. Thin worksheet, write whatever comes to mind when you think about these two words. For example, do you associate the word "success" with fat or thin? What about "funny"? How about "lazy"? You get the idea. List as many qualities as you can and notice whether you instinctively assign them to a "fat" or "thin" person.

Once you've finished, go for a walk, a swim, or a bike ride. Go to a dance class, do some yoga, or turn on some music and dance around your home. It's quite likely you'll feel a bit emotional after doing this exercise.

Later in the week, come back and read your lists. Be as objective as possible when determining whether what you've written about these words is true. How have these words affected your relationship with your body?

Fat vs. Thin

Exercise 5-1

List characteristics you associate with each word.

FAT	THIN

Lesson 14

While you may be determined to part with a few extra pounds, you may be equally determined to hold on to other things that need to go as well. You may cling to the comfort of certain foods and routines even while your deeper need may be to lighten up, take a few risks, and move in a new direction.

Every day you are given the opportunity to recreate yourself. How often do you choose the same thoughts, eat the same foods, or follow the same routine? If you want to create something different in your life, you must do something different.

The trick is to let go little by little. Instead of large leaps, start with micro-movements. Barely perceptible to others, these teeny tiny actions are absolutely essential to building up your bravery muscles.

Start by letting go of the things that don't matter so much. Say "no" to a dessert that looks fabulous but tastes like cardboard. Say "so long" to another night of sitting around watching sports and go play catch with your kids instead. Say "adios" to anything that involves organizing entire events all by yourself.

Letting go of even the smallest things can seem like a monumental request. But giving yourself the gift of a little breathing room will benefit you in unimaginable ways. For one thing, it centers you in the present and keeps you from cluttering up your life with "stuff" from the past. It also allows you to evaluate requests or question behaviors that are no longer aligned with the person you are becoming.

Putting it into practice

On this lesson's worksheet, I've included some questions for you to consider. You may want to invite some friends to join you for a discussion of the topic. Or if you're ready to dive right in on your own, get out your journal and do some exploring.

Of course, if you're not in the mood to talk about such "heavy" topics, then by all means change the subject and conjure up some side-splitting fun. The importance of humor cannot be underestimated in your effort to lighten up!

Lightening up mentally and emotionally is as beneficial as lightening up physically. Studies have shown that laughing lowers blood pressure, reduces stress hormones, increases muscle flexion, and boosts immune function by raising levels of infection-fighting T-cells. It also triggers the release of endorphins, the body's natural painkillers, and produces a general sense of well-being.

Wouldn't you prefer a good, long belly-laugh to a series of crunches? Yet most days, you're probably more likely to do the crunches than indulge in a good laugh. Without joy breaks, your body will rebel. How about rewarding yourself with a manicure, massage, or a movie marathon consisting of your favorite comedies?

Questions to Consider
Exercise 5-2

Here are a few thought starters:

1. If putting on weight served to protect or insulate you from something or someone, who or what might that be?

   _____

2. What things are not expected of you when you are out of shape or overweight or even underweight?

   _____

   _____

3. What kinds of food do you crave when you are anxious?

   _____

   _____

4. How do you handle the holidays or other special occasions?

   _____

   _____

5. Do you eat more or less when you get nervous?_____

6. Do you exercise more or less when you're stressed?_____

7. Do most of the clothes in your closet fit? _____

8. Do you limit yourself to certain styles or colors? _____

9. Are most of your clothes comfortable? _____

10. How many sizes of clothing do you have in your closet?_____

11. Do you view your body "ornamentally" or "instrumentally" — as something to be adorned and admired or something to be utilized and able to provide you with pleasure? (For more details on this concept, see Susan Kano's book, *Making Peace With Food*.)

    _____

Lesson 15

How easy was it to answer the questions posed in the last lesson? The ones I'd like you to act on immediately are the questions concerning your clothes. If you have 3 or more different sizes of clothing in your closet — commonly referred to as "fat" clothes or "skinny" clothes — it's time for some spring cleaning.

If you are now a size 12, and you're keeping a size 8 pair of jeans in your closet as an incentive, it's time to give them to your favorite charity. For you men, it may be the size 32 waist jeans that need to go. They create more guilt than inspiration. If you fit into a smaller size again, you deserve to buy yourself a new pair. In the meantime, you can't afford the cost of keeping them.

There's something deeply satisfying about giving something you no longer need to someone who does need it. As Jim Carrey in *The Grinch* said, "One person's toxic sludge is another person's potpourri." Although I wouldn't classify your clothes as toxic waste, some of the emotions you may associate with them (like guilt, shame, self-hate) come pretty close.

In my "Secrets to Stress Less Living" course we devote an entire week to clearing out clutter. I believe there is a connection between clutter control and weight control. It's worth investigating why you hold on to things (or pounds) after they've served their purpose. Is the concept of trusting yourself, the universe, God, or whatever you believe in to provide you with the strength and resources you need to succeed too scary to surrender control to at the moment?

One of my goals is to help you connect with a profound respect for life — your life, in particular. Underneath the excess weight or the compulsive dieting or exercise or general dissatisfaction is a woman or man who is overwhelmed with the burden of being less than perfect. What you need to know is you are perfect in your imperfections.

The changes you seek to make must be prompted by a respect for your body, not a disdain for it. So much more can be accomplished with compassion than criticism. Outside factors may influence how you perceive yourself, but no "body" else can determine the relationship you choose to have with the amazing vehicle that contains your spirit.

On days when you are tempted to trash your body or push it beyond its limits, remember how miraculous it is. Your heart beats without any supervision. Your digestive system is busy turning nutrients into energy. Your circulatory system is rushing blood and oxygen to wherever it is needed. Your reproductive system may even be busy creating a new life. All this without a lot of thought from you. Imagine what conscious consideration from you might do!

Putting it into practice

I realize I've been asking you to work incredibly hard and dig deeply into areas you may have preferred to avoid. In order for you not to become overwhelmed, I'm giving you permission to take a little break. I do, however, have a suggestion for your time away from the course work.

Instead of heading to warm beaches or snowy slopes, I'd like you to head to your closet. It is there that your toughest workout awaits!

Usually the closet exercise is saved for "special occasions" — namely moving. That's when your practical side takes over and determines it's better to give your clothes away rather than rent another moving van to lug them around with you. Because you are initiating a move in a new direction, this symbolic activity sends a message to your soul. You are letting go of the past and opening up to the present. (Cleaning your closets never sounded so good, did it?)

Be prepared to have an emotional attachment to your clothes. This is where a good friend or the teenager next door can be of assistance.

They will reassure you that although disco may be making a comeback, that silver-sequined, off-the-shoulder number never will. Your local playhouse or theater may have use for it though. If the clothes are clean and in good shape, donate them to a women's shelter or Goodwill.

By cleaning out your closets and leaving only fabulous clothes that fit, getting dressed becomes infinitely more appealing than staying in your pajamas all day!

Closet Cleaning Tips
Exercise 5-3

Helpful Hints

1. Take everything out of your closet. Scrub down the closet. (This is a good feng shui practice as well as a good housekeeping idea.)

2. Organize clothes into four piles: keep, discard, donate, swap or sell.
   - If you haven't worn it in a year, discard, donate, swap, or sell it.
   - If it's too tight or too big, discard, donate, swap, or sell it.
   - If it's stained or needs mending, discard it.
   - If it's no longer in fashion, discard, donate, swap, or sell it.
   - If you have duplicates of the same items, discard, donate, swap, or sell the extra items.

3. Sort the remaining clothes by season or occasion. Store in appropriate areas.

4. Use closet organizers to arrange your clothes and shoes so when you open your closet every day, only outfits that fit are available to you.

5. Congratulate yourself on freeing up enormous amounts of energy!

Chapter Six

Stretch Your Knowledge

Lesson 16

Congratulations! If you've been reading a chapter a week, journaling, and adding some form of movement to your schedule, you've long passed the 21-day mark experts say it takes to form a new habit. That means you've gone beyond the "good idea" stage to implementing the changes in your thoughts and actions that constitute the "good practice" stage.

So, how is it going? Do you think about yourself differently than you did a month ago? Do you think about eating in a different way? Does exercise appeal to you more than it did a month ago? Are you more accepting or compassionate with yourself? Do you have more energy? Do you feel more confident in your body?

Becoming aware of how, when, why, where, or with whom you eat and/or exercise often provides the catalyst for change. The key to remember is: although working through this program only takes a few months, the foundation you build here is meant to last a lifetime. Take the time necessary to build a solid foundation.

Do not be discouraged if you have not lost "X" number of pounds by now or have failed to make it through an entire hip hop class without taking a break. If you were making grand claims already, I would wonder whether they were maintainable.

Your mind thrives on a steady stream of nourishing thoughts just as your body thrives on a steady stream of nourishing foods. Feed it with equal attention and discipline.

To help you with that steady stream of nourishing thoughts, I've created a list of Body Confidence Boosters for you to copy and put around your home in places where you will see them often. Even if you are not yet able to digest this food for thought, it's important for you to be exposed to it. These life-affirming, confidence-boosting suggestions help counterbalance the subliminal negativity you're exposed to every time you pick up a magazine, turn on the television, or listen to the radio.

For even greater benefit, compose a few Body Confidence Boosters of your own. You may want to record your boosters on tape so you can hear your own voice repeat them back to you when you are struggling or feeling like you want to give up.

The most effective boosters are written in the present tense and start with the words "I am." Keep your statements positive instead of negative. For example, "I am exercising for twenty minutes every day," instead of "I don't give in to my urge to skip exercising." Allow these thoughts to nourish your body and soul.

Body Confidence Boosters

I am a person of incredible beauty and strength.

I am strong in body and soul.
My strength serves me well and helps me
define who I am and what I am capable of doing and becoming.

I radiate confidence in myself and my body.

My body responds to the increased physical demands I place upon it
by becoming stronger, more flexible, and aerobically fit.

I move easily and naturally in my body. I breathe deeply and easily
and allow life to unfold in the present moment.

I sprinkle joy throughout my activities and
enjoy a great sense of humor.

I am flexible and able to flow with life.
I can move in whatever direction is necessary.
I respond calmly to situations with clarity and focus.

I am committed to bringing forth the best
in myself and those around me.

I trust myself and my impressions, feelings, and inner wisdom.

I have purpose and great passion.
Each experience lends itself to the unfolding of my unique path.
The world anticipates and appreciates my many gifts.

I am able to balance the many facets of my life so
that I am fully present and able to enjoy each day.

As I grow stronger in my body, I allow myself to grow stronger
in my relationships with others. I express my truth and allow
myself to experience a greater range of emotions.

Movement allows my body to free itself of unnecessary stress
and tension. Movement allows my mind to free itself
of negative thoughts and familiar patterns.

Taking care of myself is the best gift I can give to others.

I am committed to bringing about positive changes in my life.
I realize these changes may take me out of comfort zone, and
I may feel frightened, frustrated, and even like a failure.
However, I am making these changes out of a deep respect
for myself and the quality of my life.

I manage the flow of my energy and recognize what gives me energy
and what zaps my energy. I can quickly recover my balance
and energy by staying centered and present.

I possess immense personal power.
I practice connecting with this
place of strength and inner guidance regularly.
I can easily tap into this place of power whenever I feel
frightened, confused, or unsettled.

I make healthy choices regarding the foods I eat,
the people I surround myself with, the work I do,
and the way I take care of my body.
I enjoy vibrant health and supportive relationships.
My work honors my creativity, intellectual and
emotional intelligence, and social skills.
My dedication to exercise rewards me with
increased energy, strength, stamina, and flexibility.

I feed my body nutritious foods and my mind nutritious thoughts.

I am fearless. I follow my fascination as it takes me to new places, introduces me to new people, and allows me become all of who I am.

I let go of habits, relationships, and situations that no longer support me. By letting go of what no longer serves me, I attract people and opportunities that support the person I am becoming.

I am open to new opportunities and experiences that allow me to exercise parts of myself that I may not have acknowledged previously.

My increasing strength, stamina, and flexibility benefit me in many practical and exciting ways.

I am committed to a path of health and well-being.
Each day I make choices that support my journey on this path.
I am committed to enjoying myself as I exercise.
I am committed to learning how different foods affect my energy level and my ability to concentrate or perform at my best.
I am committed to engaging my imagination, following my fascination, and doing things out of sheer joy.
I am committed to communicating openly and honestly with others and speaking my truth.
I am committed to using my power in an authentic way.

I honor the rhythms and cycles of my body and soul.

I respect my body's need for rest as well as movement.
I respect my soul's need for quiet time as well as companionship.
I respect the cycles of birth and death and allow for the passage of certain ideas, relationships, or careers and the emergence of new ones that acknowledge the person I am now.

I am committed to keeping my mind, body, and spirit
alive and energized.
I am willing to try new activities, learn new skills,
and meet new people.
I am willing to be patient with myself as I open to new ways of doing
things and experiencing life. I am kind and gentle with myself as
I open to the possibilities that unfold.

I am grateful for my health and the courage to continue
on this path towards wholeness.

Putting it into practice

One of the most common questions heard around the world is "what's
for dinner?" Since eating is something most of us do anywhere from
one to ten times a day, this constant question offers us unlimited choices. Yet how often do we make conscious choices that truly satisfy our
hunger?

What follows is an exercise to help you the next time someone asks,
"What do you want to eat?" Instead of the standard "I don't know,
what do you want?" reply, this worksheet encourages you to identify
the texture, taste, temperature, and temperament of your cravings.

While doing this exercise I suggest you take a few deep breaths, drop
down into your belly, and put your hand over your abdomen while you
ask yourself the questions. It might take some practice before you can
interpret your body's signals. But eventually you will be able to answer
the "what do you want to eat?" question with a definitive "fresh garden
salad, baked salmon, wild rice, and water with a lemon wedge, please."

What Nourishes Me?
Exercise 6-1

1. Am I hungry for something hot? If yes, what might I eat that is hot and nutritious?

   _____

2. Am I hungry for something cold? If yes, what might I eat that is cold and nutritious?

   _____

3. Am I hungry for something crunchy? If yes, what might I eat that is crunchy and nutritious?

   _____

4. Am I hungry for something soft? If yes, what might I eat that is soft and nutritious?

   _____

5. What color appeals to me right now? What foods of this color are available and appetizing to me?

   _____

6. Do I need something spicy or mild? Do I crave something exotic or traditional?

   _____

7. Do I want someone else to prepare it or would I prefer to make it?

   _____

8. On a scale of 1-10 (with 10 being ravenous), how hungry am I? Do I want to eat now or wait a while?

   _____

Lesson 17

What did you discover about your eating preferences? If you do this exercise often, you'll begin to recognize patterns as well as preferences. You'll also realize when you have a particular craving for one thing but try to substitute another, the craving will continue to demand your attention. If you really want something hot, but eat something cold, you may find yourself seeking out something hot to satisfy your craving, even if you are full.

Another interesting thing you may notice is that sometimes your "hunger" may not be physical at all. Maybe you hunger for quiet time? Maybe you hunger for the touch of a loved one? Maybe you hunger for some intellectual stimulation? Maybe you hunger for beautiful landscapes?

Yet, many times, it's more convenient to reach for food than ask for or seek out what you truly need. It's safer to swallow your emotions than speak out. It's easier to go for a run than go on a blind date. It takes less energy to turn on the television than to attend a lecture on something of interest. You tell yourself you "should" do this or that, but may not take a step in that direction.

Why? Is it just human nature to resist change? Possibly. It's also a matter of desire. When you truly want to do something, you figure out a way to do it. Most things are not hard to do. They are just easier not to do. When you're committed, when you've determined that what you do or don't do matters, you will find the energy to do the seemingly difficult things along the way.

Putting it into practice

The next exercise is called "Time Out." To answer these questions honestly you will need to get quiet and allow yourself some time to really explore your answers. I encourage you to ask yourself one or all of these questions on a daily basis, so you start to know what you really want or need and stop substituting things that don't satisfy you.

Time Out

Exercise 6-2

1. What do I need physically right now? What am I really hungry for? Do I want to eat a salad or shish-ka-bob ? Do I want to get some exercise? Do I want to take a nap?

_____

_____

_____

2. What do I need emotionally right now? Do I need to let off steam and anger or celebrate my accomplishments? Do I need to ask for a hug or write a letter to my congressman or congresswoman?

_____

_____

_____

3. What do I need intellectually right now? What does my mind yearn for? Do I want to go to the library? Do I want to read a book, catch a movie, or work a crossword puzzle?

_____

_____

_____

4. What do I need spiritually right now? How can I feed my soul? Do I want to feed the pigeons? Do I feel like visiting a florist and breathing in the beautiful fragrances?

_____

_____

_____

5. What do I need financially right now? Would I enjoy being generous to myself and others and treating for lunch? Or do I want a free
lunch? Do I want to buy something outrageous or put some money
in the bank?

_____

_____

_____

6. What do I need from others right now? Do I need companionship
or alone time? Do I want to smile at strangers or pretend I'm invisible? Do I feel like complimenting someone, laughing with them, or
arguing with them?

_____

_____

_____

7. What do I need from my environment right now? Do I need some
space to move around? Do I want to walk in the park or retreat to
my room and listen to soothing music? Am I moved to pick up litter
or water the plants?

_____

_____

_____

8. What do I need to feel on purpose right now? Do I need to gaze at
the clouds, call my mother, give a dog a bone, or follow up with a
client? Do I want to meditate or take a drive?

_____

_____

_____

Lesson 18

Did you discover that your hunger for other things is as insistent as your hunger for food? In a society constantly subjected to conflicting messages about food, we're encouraged to find fearlessness in a can of caffeine, develop relationships over fast food, and stretch our dollars — and our waistlines — by "super sizing" everything. No wonder we are tempted to turn to food for a fix.

Most of us don't know what it's like to go hungry. We have more than enough most of the time. We waste food, send it back until it meets our specifications, deny ourselves the right to certain foods, or splurge and then purge. We use food as a substitute for what we really crave.

We've lost touch with our real hunger. Instead of honoring it as the source of energy that sustains our life, food has become the enemy. It's the barrier that stands between us and our ideal. After all, if we could just stop eating so much, maybe we could finally lose those extra pounds and be happy. Or not. I hope you've learned by now that the solution is not nearly that simple.

You may have a healthy respect for food and are conscious of the food you choose from conception to consumption. However, it's important to understand the mentality of the culture you are a part of and how it influences your choices.

Putting it into practice

During the first four chapters, I asked you to engage in aerobic activities such as walking or biking or swimming. How are you doing with this? Are you able to walk longer or farther than before? Are you experiencing an increase in your energy level?

Now I'd like you to add another essential component to your fitness routine — stretching. There are many classes devoted to various types of flexibility training. If classes are not your thing, can you discover ways to stretch at your desk, at home, or while waiting in line?

Experiment with stretching your mind, stretching a dollar, stretching your limits, stretching your comfort zone, etc. Flexibility can be practiced in all kinds of arenas.

Increasing Flexibility
Exercise 6-3

1. How could I benefit from developing more flexibility in my life?

   _____

   _____

2. What activities would be easier to perform if I were more flexible?

   _____

3. What situations might flow more smoothly if my attitude were more flexible?

   _____

4. Do I view being flexible as negative or positive? _____

5. What negative experiences do I associate with being flexible?

   _____

6. Who personifies flexibility to me? _____

7. What would being more flexible look and feel like to me?

   _____

8. Do I believe I could benefit from becoming more flexible? ____

9. If so, what activities am I willing to commit to so I can increase my flexibility?

   _____

10. How much time am I willing to devote to increasing my flexibility?

   _____

11. How important is it for me to be flexible?

   _____

12. When was the last time I exhibited my flexibility?

   _____

Chapter Seven

Feed Your Curiosity

Lesson 19

One day I caught the end of a cooking show on television and heard the host proclaim, "Any meal you don't remember is merely fast food." It made sense to me.

How many times do you rush through meals to get on to something more important? Isn't nourishing yourself an equally important activity? I'm not suggesting every meal become an obsession or food become the focus of your entire day. I am suggesting that each meal deserves your acknowledgement and conscious consideration. Even the sorriest excuse for a sandwich requires effort on someone's part to offer sustenance.

Whether you're limited by time, budget, ability, or creativity, you can still eat well if you so desire. Given the fact that eating is something you will do the rest of your life, it makes sense to spend a little time figuring out what you like, what you don't like, what gives you energy, what depletes your energy, etc.

The subject of nutrition could easily consume the entire book. Since it is not my area of expertise but it is an important component of Body Confidence, I'll give you a very brief overview of the subject.

Basic nutrition is pretty straightforward. A lot of damage has been done by making nutrition much more complicated or confusing than it needs to be. Here is the way I understand it. All foods are made up of various combinations of the six basic nutrients: carbohydrates, fats, proteins, vitamins, minerals, and water. Most foods have some of all the nutrients, just in different percentages. Since no single food can supply all the nutrients in the amounts you need, it's best to eat a variety of foods.

Carbohydrates are a primary source of energy for the cells in your body — brain cells, muscle cells, etc. The primary purpose of fat is energy production. Proteins provide the structure for the many cells and tissues in the body. They are also used in the immune system, to transport vital elements in the bloodstream, and to make up many of the hormones. Vitamins and minerals are essential for the proper working of the body's multitude of functions. And finally, water is necessary to maintenance of proper body temperature and helps transport nutrients and waste products in and out of cells.

Where things get confusing is trying to figure out which foods contain which nutrients and how much of these foods you need on a daily basis. The good news is, if you have an Internet connection, much of this information can be found at your fingertips.

The USDA has come out with a new pyramid designed to remind consumers to make healthy food choice and be active every day. To personalize the plan and find out what your specific dietary and exercise needs are visit www.mypyramid.gov.

Of course there are many sources of information you may wish to explore and I encourage you to look at more than one source. Your best bet, if you have the budget, may be to meet with a certified nutritionist who can help you sift through the information you've compiled and translate it into a plan that works for you based on your particular needs.

Putting it into practice

Many times meals become an unconscious act of feeding ourselves everything but the nourishment our bodies are truly craving. How many times have you sat down to eat a meal while simultaneously attempting to catch the latest news on the television, radio, or newspaper and from your children, spouse, roommate, or pet? With all that commotion, can you even remember what you ate — let alone what it tasted like?

This exercise asks you to think about the last meal you truly enjoyed and felt nourished by. We are fed on many levels, and often find ourselves nourished or famished by the "nutrients" we take in. Proper nutrition consists not only of what we eat, but how, when, where, with whom, and why we eat. By doing this exercise, you may begin to recognize what truly nourishes you. Bon appetit!

The Last Supper
Exercise 7-1

The last meal I truly enjoyed was _____

_____

I ate the meal at (where) _____

and shared it with _____

The meal was prepared by _____

The meal consisted of _____

_____

_____

_____

The meal lasted _____

What I remember most about the atmosphere was (consider the lights/sound/smells, etc.)

_____

_____

I felt _____

_____

_____

What nourished me most was _____

_____

_____

_____

Lesson 20

You face a tough challenge in making appropriate choices that provide the nutrition you need because the food industry often employs misleading marketing devices in order to increase sales. By using catchwords and phrases such as "100% Natural," "Nothing Artificial," "Fortified," "Wheat Bread," "Cholesterol Free," and "Lite," advertisers try to convince consumers that their product is a better nutritional choice than it truly is.

For example, "lite" can refer to the color of something as opposed to any reduced caloric content. Something that is "100% Natural" can contain a lot of natural sugar. Unless 100% whole wheat is listed as the main ingredient, "wheat bread" is no different than white bread.

It pays to read the labels on the foods you buy. You may not be getting what you think you are. A label that states a certain food has reduced fat or reduced sodium means that the amount of fat or sodium has been reduced by 25% from the original product. This might imply that the food is low in fat or sodium, but it doesn't mean that it really is.

Pay attention to the serving size as well. Don't assume an item contains only one serving just because the package is small. For example, if you eat a bag of pretzels from a vending machine, you may find that it contains two or three servings. You will need to multiply the numbers by two or three to figure out how many calories and the amount of sodium and other nutrients you are consuming if you eat the whole bag.

Even though you may be using less sugar in your home, the food industry is using more of it in processed foods. As Susan Kano points out in her book, *Making Peace with Food*, "food producers add some form of simple sugar to most beverages, breads, cereals, crackers, canned foods, flavored yogurt, fast-food hamburgers and hundreds of other common foods."

There are several names for sugar: corn syrup, sucrose, glucose, dextrose, maltose, lactose, fructose, honey, and molasses. Most labels don't list the amounts of these ingredients, so you can only get a vague idea of how much sugar you consume.

Nutritionists and other health professionals urge us to limit our diet to fresh fruits, vegetables, legumes, and whole grains while the food industry and media encourage us to eat many prepared foods — most of which contain simple sugars, processed grains, and a lot of fat.

The typical American diet is not a healthy one. Making nutritious choices requires a mix of education, discipline, and desire. Many food manufacturers count on you to choose convenience over curiosity or quality. Feed your curiosity and find out what you are putting into your body.

Putting it into practice

As you prepare your meals today, take a moment to review the nutritional content of the foods you eat. Then ask yourself the following questions.

The Foods You Choose
Exercise 7-2

1. Why did I choose these foods?

_____

_____

2. How much influence did advertising have on my decision?

_____

_____

3. How much influence did taste or individual preference have on my choice?

_____

_____

4. How much influence did nutritional content exert on my decision?

_____

_____

5. Was I misled by any advertising about this product?

_____

_____

6. What can I learn from reading the label?

_____

_____

7. Are there additional ingredients in this product that seem un-necessary?

_____

_____

8. How many suggested servings does this product provide? _____

Lesson 21

Okay, now that I've exposed the "evils" of the food industry and the media, let me switch gears. I'd like to celebrate our freedom of choice (even if those choices can be overwhelming) and appreciate the abundance of available food sources.

In America most of us can buy fresh fruits and vegetables regardless of the season. Our grocery store shelves are stocked with a variety of foods and often two or three different brands of every item. I've never known it to be any different. But I do know this is not the case for many people.

I have been blessed. I grew up on a farm where apples, pears, sweet corn, green beans, peas, tomatoes, cucumbers, strawberries, watermelon, cantaloupe, pumpkins, etc. were mine for the picking. I'll never forget the exquisite taste of an apple picked from our very own tree or the sweetness of corn plucked and shucked from the field. There was a sense of connection with the source that added to the appreciation of the food.

Despite the desire for quick and easy meals that come in a box and require little more than minimal attention, there is an art to preparing, presenting, and partaking in a meal that satisfies the soul as much as the stomach. This shouldn't be overlooked.

A dear friend illustrated this art when I was leaving a life I loved in Santa Fe to return to my family farm in Illinois and an unforeseen future. She spent an entire weekend preparing scrumptious foods to serve at my farewell dinner. I was nourished for many days to come by that meal.

I'm sure you, too, have tales of love and support, struggles and strife shared over meals you'll never forget. Shortly after returning to the farm, I went to a luncheon at one of the local churches. I remember thinking, "These are the foods from my childhood." In front of me were various salads, casseroles, desserts, and all kinds of food I had never made for myself. Instantly I was transported back in time.

Foods and their accompanying smells have an amazing way of weaving life stories together. Their magical qualities have inspired more than a few books and films. My hope is that you can give up constant calorie counting for the consistent counting of your blessings and allow the sensuous experience of eating to nourish your body and soul.

Putting it into practice

In our effort to analyze, criticize, or rationalize our food choices we often forget to recognize our great fortune in simply having enough to eat. This week as you partake of your meals, take a moment to acknowledge the source of your food, the people who participated in preparing it, and the nourishment it is providing. This does not have to be a formal prayer, just a conscious awareness.

Slow down while you eat. Instead of reading the paper, watching the television, or otherwise "multitasking," just eat. Notice the texture, temperature, and taste of your food. Put your silverware down between bites. Don't entertain thoughts of seconds until you've first digested what's in front of you. Allow yourself to eat as much as you want as long as you are in touch with your real needs.

Often you are tempted to eat much more than you need because you are distracted. If there is fast-paced music playing or high-action drama on the television screen, you will probably eat faster and eat more than if you were paying attention to the meal itself. Notice how, when, where, and with whom you usually eat and see if you can make some adjustments.

Those who have diabetes or other chronic conditions requiring close attention to diet can attest to the importance of planning. Having the right kinds of food available when you need them plays a huge part in maintaining your health on a daily basis.

Although I'm not much of a cook and I tend to avoid grocery shopping, I have discovered that I make better choices about what I eat when I take the time to plan for my meals. Stocking the refrigerator and pantry with nutritious foods is much easier to do on a full stomach than when I'm hungry, tired, or crabby.

For those of you with families, the task becomes even more challenging. You may be operating under several conditions that conspire against you: limited time, limited budget, limited energy, fussy eaters, etc. Some days you may have to compromise on optimal nutritional value in order to achieve peace of mind.

The following food planning guide was inspired by Body Confidence graduate, Linda Brakeall. You may want to use it to come up with your next shopping list.

Food Planning Guide
Exercise 7-3

Who knows better than you how your body works and responds?

Morning

A good breakfast that will keep me going until lunch is:

_____

When I eat _____ for breakfast, I feel sluggish.

When I eat _____ for breakfast, I feel energetic.

I feel better when for breakfast I eat:

_____ protein (eggs, cheese, meat, fish)

_____ starchy foods (breads, cereals, bagels)

_____ fruits

Foods I like for breakfast: _____

_____

Understanding that a good breakfast is a positive start for my day, here are three good breakfasts for me:

1. _____

2. _____

3. _____

On days I don't have time for breakfast, a healthy choice I can grab and eat on the run is:

_____

A good mid-morning snack for me would be:

_____

Mid-Day

I'm usually ready for lunch by _____

If I eat a big lunch, in the afternoon I feel _____

If I eat a small lunch, in the afternoon I feel _____

If I don't eat lunch at all, in the afternoon I feel _____

I feel better when for lunch I eat:

_____ protein (eggs, cheese, meat, fish)

_____ starchy foods (breads, cereals, bagels)

_____ fruits

Foods I like for lunch: _____

_____

Understanding that a good lunch keeps me well nourished and pro-
ductive, here are three good lunches for me:

1. _____

2. _____

3._____

On days I don't have time for lunch, a healthy choice I can grab and
eat on the run is:

_____

A good mid-afternoon snack for me would be:

_____

Evening

I'm usually ready for dinner by _____

If I eat a big dinner, I feel _____

If I eat a small dinner, I feel _____

If I don't eat dinner at all, I feel _____

I feel better when for dinner I eat:

_____ protein (eggs, cheese, meat, fish)

_____ starchy foods (breads, cereals, bagels)

_____ fruits

Foods I like for dinner: _____

_____

Understanding that a good dinner keeps me well nourished, and prevents after-dinner mischief, here are three good dinners for me:

1. _____

2. _____

3. _____

On days I don't have time for dinner, a healthy choice I can grab and eat on the run is:

_____

A good after-dinner snack for me would be:

_____

Chapter Eight

Build Your Personal Power

Lesson 22

Part of Body Confidence comes from knowing how your body will react to any number of variables. In the past couple of chapters you been noticing how the foods you choose affect your health. Now it's time to notice how your thoughts and beliefs impact your health, specifically your stress level.

Where your mind goes, your body is likely to follow. Regardless of what's really going on, your body will respond to your mind's interpretation. If that interpretation is one that threatens your well-being, it automatically sets a series of physiological responses in motion.

Stored sugars and fats are released into the blood stream to provide quick energy. Digestion ceases so that more blood is available to the brain and muscles. Muscles tense in preparation for action. Pupils dilate, and your sense of smell and hearing become more acute. Perspiration increases to help reduce your body temperature. Your breathing rate increases to provide more oxygen to the blood. Your heart beats faster to supply more blood to the muscles.

Within moments, your body is ready, willing, and able to fight for your life. Yet how often is that truly necessary? How many times is your body all stressed out with nowhere to go? How many times does that lack of real direction lead you to the kitchen to find comfort in chips, cookies, cakes, colas, or chocolate? Or drive you to exercise past the point of exhaustion?

Stress usually leaves you feeling out of control. There are many ways to regain your sense of control and find your center. In this chapter, I'll share a few stress reducing strategies that can help you restore your personal power. But first, let's determine how stress shows up in your life.

Putting it into practice

Here are a few exercises to get you thinking about how you handle stress and how it shows up in your body.

All Stressed Out
Exercise 8-1

1. When I'm stressed out I eat more _____, less _____, or about the same _____ as I normally do.

2. When I'm stressed out I exercise more _____, less _____, or about the same _____ as I normally do.

3. When I'm stressed out I drink more _____, less _____, or about the same _____ as I normally do.

4. When I'm stressed out I sleep more _____, less _____, or about the same _____ as I normally do.

5. My worst coping strategy for handling stress is _____

   _____

6. My best coping strategy for handling stress is _____

   _____

7. Stress shows up in my body as _____

   _____

8. Stress shows up in my relationships as _____

   _____

9. When I'm stressed out I crave _____

   _____

10. What stresses me out the most in my daily life is _____

    _____

11. The one thing I could do to relieve most of my stress is_____

    _____

12. I believe I have the power _____ am powerless _____ to make the changes necessary to reduce my stress level.

I Feel It Here
Exercise 8-1a

1. What am I feeling? _____

_____

2. What is underneath this feeling? _____

_____

3. How does this affect my body? Where am I carrying tension?

_____

_____

4. How is this impacting my life right now? Is it pulling my attention away from the present moment?

_____

_____

5. When did this feeling start? What happened and what did I tell myself about what happened?

_____

_____

6. Was I expecting something of someone? Did I make some false assumptions?

_____

_____

7. Am I able to work through the uncomfortable feelings?

_____

8. What can I do in the future to create a different outcome?

_____

_____

Lesson 23

It can start off innocently enough. You misplace your car keys or ac-
cidentally feed the fish dog food instead of tropical mix and shrimp
pellets. Suddenly annoying events begin to gather momentum. You set
your briefcase down on your child's breakfast as you discover a tooth-
paste stain on your favorite shirt. Before you can count to ten, a full-
blown meltdown is in process.

You may feel your blood pressure rise simply reading this. Maybe because it's happened to you or someone in your household more times
than you care to remember. Or you may shrug it off as an opportunity
to celebrate your starring role in the theater of the absurd.

To stress or not to stress — that is the question. Yet how many times
do you even consider it a choice? After all, who wouldn't seek solace in
pecan praline ice cream or some other soothing substance after a day
of miscommunications, missed appointments, and mismanagement
all around?

You wouldn't. Because you have an arsenal of effective coping skills,
you'd head to the nearest park and walk off your worries. Or you might
surrender to the situation and allow a massage therapist to coax the
tension out of your body. Or you put on your gardening gloves and do
some serious digging, allowing the earth to absorb your anxiety and
return you to your center.

The more you can involve your body in releasing your stress, the better. Whether it be a solitary swim, a game of racquetball, or a good cry,
your body needs an outlet for the inner tension. When neurotransmit-
ters like adrenaline, norepinephrine, dopamine, and additional hormones are released into the blood stream, ready to be deployed, and
then discover their mission is aborted, eventually they stop working

for you and start working against you.

You have probably experienced the fight or flight response hard-wired into your body. Your first response may be to lash out, argue, throw something, or create a scene. Perhaps the urge to bolt overtakes you the moment someone asks you to say a few words at your child's recital or after you've been summoned into the boss's office for no apparent reason or when you get a call from your doctor's office. Or possibly you are so stunned you simply freeze, like a deer caught in the headlights.

The fourth option — and often the best — is to flow. Where fighting, fleeing, or freezing are automatic responses, flowing is a learned response and requires regular practice to master. Flowing implies that you've gotten enough control over your mind to slow down the stress response in your body. This allows you to center yourself in the present moment and act from a place of power instead of fear.

Arriving at this outcome takes practice. Any number of disciplines can help you achieve more flow in your life. Yoga, martial arts, meditation, and mindfulness practices may help you become aware of your breathing and the role it plays in helping you get centered. Or maybe running, cycling, swimming, or skiing work best for you.

Once you choose your method, the real work begins. Mastering any discipline takes time, commitment, and effort. However, the more you flow in response to stress, the more you'll want to cultivate it in all areas of your life.

Connecting with your breath is a great way to calm yourself and flow with events. When you're stressed, you tend to take short, shallow gulps of air. When your thoughts are racing, your body follows suit. However, if you can slow down your breathing, you can slow down your thoughts enough to question their validity.

Try this. Place one hand over your belly and the other on your chest. Now take a nice, deep breath. Which hand moved first? If you're like most people, it was probably the hand over your chest. In belly breathing or diaphragmatic breathing, the goal is to make the hand over your belly move first, indicating the breath has found its way into the lower lungs. If you are a singer, you may have mastered this technique in order to get the most out of your voice.

I've asked you to notice all kinds of things during this course from what, when, where, why, and how you exercise, eat, and think to how you breathe. Gaining awareness of your current behavior is essential to any behavioral change program whether it be losing weight or reducing stress.

Today, pay attention to your breathing. Notice how it changes throughout the day during different activities and with different people and in different situations. Take a few minutes throughout the day to pay attention to the in breath, the out breath, and the space in between breaths.

What follows is a script for a guided visualization you can use to relax and reconnect with your breath in as little as 3–5 minutes.

Relaxation Visualization

- Sit comfortably in an open body position (nothing crossed) and close your eyes.

- Take a deep breath and repeat the word "relax" to yourself 3 times, visualizing the word on the inside of your eyelids.

- Take a second deep breath and tell yourself to slow the tempo of your thoughts and quiet your mind.

- A third deep breath and imagine you are in the most calm, relaxing place you have ever been. Place yourself within that scene and see what you saw, hear what you heard, smell any scents present.

- After several seconds, draw your attention to your scalp and allow it to completely and totally RELAX.

- In the same manner, work your way down through your body, area by area, to your toes.

- Then do a final scan of your body for any lingering tightness or stress and direct it to drain out through your feet into the ground.

- Say to yourself the following affirmations:

  I radiate vitality and robust well-being.

  I am fully prepared and equipped to handle whatever I face today.

  I am entitled to a life of my own design.

- Take another deep breath. Slowly bring your awareness back to present time and open your eyes.

Putting it into practice

In order to track down the sources of your stress and become aware of your typical response, you'll need to do a little detective work. For the next seven days, jot down the stress producers you encounter throughout your day. Each time you feel stressed, tense, or anxious, record the cause and the effects.

Stress Detector
Exercise 8-2

1. When did the stressful event happen (date and time)?

_____

2. Where were you? _____

_____

3. What happened? _____

_____

_____

4. Who was involved? _____

_____

5. What precipitated the event?_____

_____

6. How stressed were you (on a scale of 1–10)? _____

7. How did you handle it?_____

_____

_____

8. Why do you think it happened? _____

_____

_____

After recording your "stress incidents" for seven days, you'll probably start to see some patterns emerge. Who tends to push your buttons — kids, co-workers, clients? What environment is most stressful for you — meetings, mornings before work, social obligations? When do you tend to lose it — when you're hungry, angry, lonely, tired, or pre-occupied with something else?

Lesson 24

How much of your stress stems from having too much to do in too little time? Do you tell yourself if you had more time you'd prepare nutritious meals, exercise more, enjoy yourself more, or do any number of things you may not be doing now?

In my experience, unless I can handle what I've got, more of it only leads to bigger challenges. I don't believe more time is the answer. Making the most of the time available is. As you set about changing habits, patterns, and beliefs that have been a lifetime in the making, give yourself plenty of breathing room and allow for errors.

Instead of adding to your already full schedule, what might you take away from it? What activities are just adding the buzz to your busyness but not really providing you with any extra energy or enhancing your life in some way? Where might you recover pockets of time and energy that can be used to create the microscopic changes that eventually allow the monumental ones to occur?

For me, reducing my stress level is a two-fold process. One is practicing techniques that allow me to center myself physically and slow down the internal noise. This might include stretching, meditating, lifting weights, or taking my dog for a long walk.

The other is a spiritual surrender that involves believing in my own ability to handle whatever happens. This may include calling upon a higher power for assistance or asking for help from others when I need it.

The best stress-reducing strategy I know is a paradoxical one. It requires taking control and surrendering at the same time. You need to take control of your thoughts and reactions but surrender your perceived control of events, people, or outcomes.

Putting it into practice

This week you're going to add strength training to your fitness routine. Yes, you're adding "stress" to your muscles in order to solicit their best response.

While weight work at the gym might be the most effective way to build your strength, do not discount the many ways you can work a little strength training into your day. Carrying meeting minutes from your desk to the conference room requires strength. Lugging groceries from the store to your car to your house requires strength. Lifting your kids requires strength. Moving wet laundry from the wash machine to the clothesline requires strength. Take advantage of every opportunity you encounter to use your strength.

In her book, *A Woman's Book of Strength*, Karen Andes says, "At the center of resistance work is discomfort — one reason why so many avoid it. The discomfort needn't be extreme or prolonged. But it's necessary to train ourselves to stay in it, if only for a moment, because this is the moment of both conflict and opportunity."

Strength training is hard work. It requires us to awaken the active, outgoing, yang forces within ourselves instead of succumbing to the soft, inward yin forces that prefer a long soak in a hot tub.

There is no doubt that finding a form of exercise you like will increase your likelihood of sticking with it. You may prefer "soft" forms of exercise, such as tai chi, yoga, or walking, rather than "hard" forms, such as weight lifting, running, or tennis. By adding softness to a hard workout or difficulty to a soft workout you will enhance your overall fitness level.

For example, tai chi masters also possess amazing strength. They can throw people across a room with their invisible "soft" power. Weight lifters have to hold a moment of stillness at the bottom of a movement to gather their power and create a fluid force.

Although I encourage you to listen to your body for clues as to what type of exercise you need, do not be fooled by mental fatigue. Have you ever thought you were too tired to exercise only to find yourself totally rejuvenated by a friend's invitation to dinner?

Some days simply demand the resistance a good weight or water workout provides. Other days we need the surrender of a restorative yoga class or a long walk in the woods. Experiment with your preferences. Stop in the middle of your walk and throw a few punches or karate kicks. Pause in the middle of your weight work to stretch and breathe deeply and slowly. This will not only add variety but build balance into your workout.

What follows are a few questions for you to answer regarding strength.

Becoming Strong
Exercise 8-3

1. How could I benefit from developing more strength in my life?

   _____

2. What activities would be easier if I were physically stronger?

   _____

3. What relationships would be easier to negotiate if I were emotionally stronger?

   _____

4. Do I view being strong as negative or positive? _____

5. What negative experiences do I associate with being strong?

   _____

6. Who personifies strength to me? _____

7. What would being stronger look and feel like to me?

   _____

8. Do I believe I could benefit from becoming stronger? _____

9. If so, what strength-building activities will I commit to?

   _____

10. What actions will I take to increase my emotional strength?

    _____

11. How much time will I devote to increasing my strength?

    _____

12. When was the last time I exhibited my strength? _____

13. How does being strong help me to define who I am to myself and others?

    _____

14. How does it feel to assert my personal power? _____

    _____

Chapter Nine

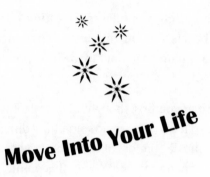

Move Into Your Life

Lesson 25

Part of experiencing Body Confidence is creating a strong enough body to back up your beliefs. Finding the courage to change any part of your life often depends on one decision, made in a moment of strength, to commit to yourself.

Think back to when you first thought about reading this book. Some part of you decided it was time to do something different. Some part of you pushed past the discomfort of what you might have to do or what you might have to change and got you to this point.

It was no small commitment on your part. Have you acknowledged that? Have you noticed the many small changes that have occurred as you have been working through this book?

You have preferences in how and when you like to move, what and when you like to eat, with whom you like to your spend time, and where you like to go. Are you more aware of them now?

When you recognize your own rhythm and move with it, you begin to move more gracefully through life. When you are forced to move to an imposed rhythm, things don't go as smoothly.

During this book, you may have become aware of an underlying rhythm similar to a heartbeat. Beat-beat-pause. Beat-beat-pause. Try something new. Relax. Try it again. Regroup. Think about it this way. Reflect. Try a different approach. Rejoice!

A few years ago I asked the artist-in-residence (a talented musician) at our local school to play live music for my exercise class. Then I invited the community to join us in a drumming circle.

The musician invited each of us to pick an instrument to play in the drumming circle. There were makeshift drums, flutes, shakers, cow-bells, even a dijeridoo or two. We each learned a particular rhythm for our instrument.

Then came the challenge of maintaining that rhythm while everyone else joined in with theirs. The initial cacophony of sounds was comical. But once we felt the rhythm, we quickly created something quite cool. It was as if each of us understood our part in the whole, if only for a few moments.

I've worked solo for a large part of my life. Although this allows me a great deal of freedom, some accomplishments require a team, a tribe, or collaborators. This book is one of them.

Just as each person contributed his or her sound to our drumming circle, you are contributing your voice to the Body Confidence process. Whether you have emailed me through the website, worked through this alone, or are part of a group, I do feel and appreciate your unique rhythm.

Putting it into practice

How often do you find yourself humming, singing, or whistling dur-ing the day? This is a very different question than how often do you find yourself sighing, groaning, or grunting. Although technically all of these are sounds, they convey completely different emotions.

My niece always has a song in her head. Mention the word library and out comes the "I'm going down to the library, picking out a book, check it in, check it out" song. After a few days with her, I start making up songs to accompany my activities.

Some time today, exercise your vocal chords. Belt out a Broadway tune, chant a mantra, or hum a hymn. If you feel inhibited about this, sing in the shower or late at night in your car in a neighboring village.

Invoke the spirit of music into your space today. Really feel your rhythm and allow your body to be transported by music. A colleague of mine, Suzanne Falter-Barns, has written wonderful books on finding and expressing your joy. She says, "You can't move others unless you yourself are moved first."

Most of us are moved by music. I know when I teach an early morning exercise class, I feel like I'm sleepwalking until I turn on the music. Then my whole being comes to life as the music moves, animates, and inspires us.

I've Got the Music in Me
Exercise 9-1

1. What music do you like to listen to in order to relax?

_____

2. What music motivates you to move and energizes you?

_____

3. What music helps you focus and think clearly?

_____

4. What music makes you feel like a kid again?

_____

5. What music makes you feel romantic?

_____

6. What's your favorite song?

_____

7. Who's your favorite artist or group?

_____

8. Is music important in your daily activities?

_____

9. What song could be the theme song for your life?

_____

10. What song do you rely on to catapult you into action?

_____

11. What song do you listen to when you need a good cry?

_____

Lesson 26

There comes a time when you realize you can only be yourself. Attempting to be anyone else robs the world of your unique contribution. Attempting to look or act like someone else strips you of your own beauty.

Yet being yourself isn't always easy. When you're encouraged to look, think, act, and feel like everyone else, being yourself becomes an act of courage.

By now, I hope you've defined what Body Confidence means to you. I also hope you have the thrill of experiencing it as part of your new reality.

Sometimes as people get older, they get weighed down by responsibilities, obligations, expectations, and accumulations. A heaviness can set in when they realize certain dreams may not be realized. This resignation can show up in their body posture just as playing a certain role in life may manifest itself in a particular look.

For example, I have a friend who has been playing out the warrior archetype in many ways, but specifically by creating a kind of body armor through years and years of weight lifting. His muscles have formed a protective suit that serves to shield him from physical or emotional attack. Although this secures his safety on some level, it also severs him from his vulnerability and seldom allows him to love deeply or feel profoundly.

I also know people who are very rigid in their thinking and need to have a lot of structure in their lives. If they show up in class, their primary challenge is flexibility. When they allow themselves to regularly stretch their bodies, I find their posture and firm grip on reality relaxes a bit as well.

What might the shape of your body reveal about the role(s) you play? Do you have the long, lean look of a huntress? How about the broad, bold build of a lumberjack? Do you have shoulders of a swimmer, the legs of a dancer, the waist of a belly dancer, the arms of an archer?

If you honestly don't know, ask someone close to you to describe your "look." It may come as a surprise to you that others see you differently than you see yourself. And yet they often see the "perfection" in you that you overlook.

Putting it into practice

Just for fun, gather a group of friends together with the intent of discovering what archetypes (universally recognized characters such as hero, warrior, victim, child, princess, etc.) are playing out in your life through your body posture.

Remember back in Chapter One when I suggested you are always broadcasting a message — usually about your current emotional state — by the way you walk, talk, or hold yourself? Here is your chance to experiment with different postures and discover how they affect your emotional state.

For example, notice the way you are sitting. Are your legs crossed, arms folded, shoulders hunched? If so, uncross your legs and arms, sit straight and take a deep breath. Notice the effect opening up your body has on your ability to take in new information.

If you are feeling sluggish, move yourself into the position or stance you take when you are energized, filled with purpose, or excited to do something. See if just by moving your body into a different posture you can influence your emotional state.

Are You My Archetype?
Exercise 9-2

1. The archetype(s) that shows up most frequently in my life is:

_____

_____

2. The physical characteristics of this archetype are:

_____

_____

3. The way this archetype or character moves is:

_____

_____

4. This character shows up most often when I am feeling:

_____

5. It might be interesting to take on the characteristics of these other archetypes:

_____

_____

6. Some activities that could help me move in different ways than I am used to are:

_____

_____

_____

_____

Lesson 27

In my exercise classes I am constantly encouraging my students to blossom — to open up to their whole selves and full life. Now I am encouraging you to do the same.

As participants and readers confide their successes and setbacks with me, I am aware that achieving Body Confidence is an ongoing process rather than a final destination. Your strength, your flexibility, your weight, your energy level, your courage, and your attitude are up for negotiation every day. You must decide daily what you will commit to.

As your inner changes manifest into outer changes and the rest of the world starts to pay attention, do not lose sight of all the factors that contribute to your new found Body Confidence. While the world may comment on your awesome arms, buns of steel, super strength, or amazing endurance, you know these outer changes are a direct reflection of the inner changes you've made.

When your mind, body, spirit, and emotions align, you have access to an incredible well of power. Unleashing your wellpower, as opposed to exerting your willpower, allows you to move into the life you deserve and desire.

The whole idea of Body Confidence was inspired by my struggle to feel safe and at home in my body. Yes, I admit to you now, more than a few of my therapy sessions have been devoted to body image.

Before anyone knew what anorexia was, I was suffering from it. From ages 14–17, I starved myself for reasons that are inexplicable to me now. Fortunately, though no information was available at the time, I "recovered" relatively quickly. My menstrual cycles eventually returned, my body filled out, and I masked my depression by exercising enough not to notice. Still the battle of the bulge waged on. It just went underground.

It wasn't until I returned to Illinois where my weight issues began and decided to write this book that I realized "recovery" is a lifelong process. I resisted writing a couple of the lessons because they hit a little too close to home. But by writing them, I began to heal wounds I didn't know still existed.

During one particular session of a body-based therapy called Synergy, I unearthed the shame I felt for not being a "petite flower." With the help of my therapist, who confided her own struggle with anorexia, I discovered a new way to view myself. I decided to see myself as a sunflower!

Sunflowers are big, bold, bodacious, and beautiful. For a sunflower to be small and delicate would be a loss to the world of flowers. When I left that session, I suddenly noticed sunflowers everywhere. It's okay to take up space, get some attention, and strut your stuff. It might just encourage others to do the same. To, in essence, blossom!

At this point in my life I am blessed with excellent health. I'm not lighter, leaner, stronger, or more flexible than I have been at other points in my life. But I do belong in my body. I appreciate all it does for me. As Belleruth Naparstek says in her guided imagery tape, my body truly is "my oldest friend, my greatest companion."

I also accept that this is the body I have been given to work with, learn from, and teach through. If I never had to worry about my weight or feel any anguish about my body, I wouldn't have been able to write this book from a place of authenticity.

What follows is a Venn diagram I designed to illustrate the influence various fitness components have on each other and your life as a whole. I originally called this process TransforMotion because I saw it as a way of transforming your life through motion of the mind, body, and spirit. Now I consider it one of the many ways to illustrate Body Confidence.

TransforMotion
©2006 Penny Plautz

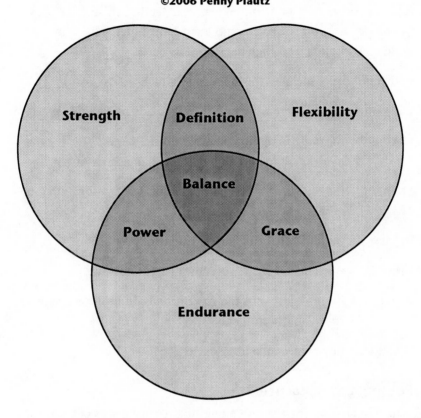

Here's how I like to explain it. When we combine strength and endurance training, we come to know our power: the depth of our courage and
resilience and our willingness to commit and persist. When we combine
flexibility and endurance training, we come to know grace: how to en-
dure endless change, flow with life, and move at what Christina Baldwin
calls, "the pace of guidance." When we combine flexibility and strength,
we define our bodies and our lives: we learn to work through our resistance, establish boundaries, and allow for emptiness. Somewhere in the
center of it all is the point of balance — different for each of us — maybe
more to the left or right, more inwardly or outwardly focused. Energy

flows into and out of this core, creating the motion that transforms our mind, body, and spirit. Although in theory, it's possible to separate the factors in order to focus on one at a time, in truth, a change in one area influences all the others. Each component contributes to the whole, rendering the whole greater than the sum of its parts.

Body Confidence includes the following characteristics:

Endurance the ability to withstand adversity or stress; lasting power

Flexibility the range of motion possible around a joint; a ready capacity to adapt to new, different, or changing requirements

Strength the capacity for exertion or endurance; a strong attribute or inherent asset

Balance the ability to bring into harmony or proportion

Grace ease and suppleness of movement or bearing

Power the physical, mental, or spiritual ability to act; energy, spirit, ability, influence

Definition: distinctness of outline or detail

Putting it into practice

What kind of flower are you? A beautiful garden consists of many varieties — each delighted to contribute its unique beauty. An iris doesn't wish to be a pansy nor a rose ache to be a tulip. In my exercise classes we give ourselves flower names to remind ourselves to open to our inherent beauty. I invite you to do the same. You might even want to do a little research on flowers and learn about their healing properties, what environments they grow best in, and what their outstanding features are. I have listed a few resources for this in the Group Resources section.

Why not come up with your own definition of Body Confidence and make a Venn diagram to illustrate it? You can do so on the following page.

Body Confidence from the Inside Out
Venn Diagram
Exercise 9-3

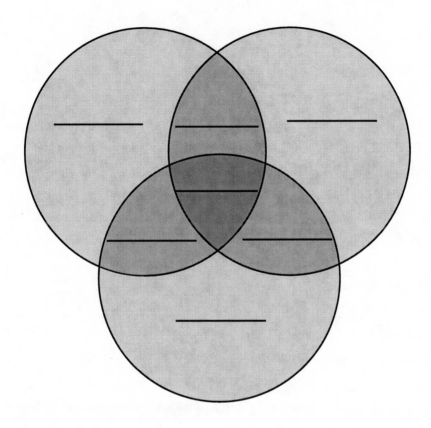

Chapter Ten

Body Confidence in the Bedroom, the Boardroom, & Beyond

Lesson 28

Despite all the other ways of measuring Body Confidence, for some of us the real test lies in our ability to walk around a water park wearing only our swimming suits or allow our naked selves to be seen by another person in a brightly lit bedroom. It's hard to imagine that anyone could overlook the obvious physical flaws that are so apparent to us, but love looks with soft eyes and seldom sees imperfections as the evil enemy we do.

It's hard to imagine that someone else might find the curve of our bellies or the softness of our skin more of a turn-on than the turn-off we believe the stretch marks on our breasts, the cellulite on our thighs, or the excess skin under our arms to be.

I'm hoping by now you've developed the inner strength and conviction that your worth can not be determined by anyone else's standards. What started out as a tiny pilot light is now ablaze with the beauty you are radiating from within. And like bees to honey, this self-confidence is attracting all kinds of opportunities to you — from the bedroom to the boardroom and beyond.

If you think about the people you most admire most and list the qualities that make them so special, I'm betting they are not things like "sex appeal," or "she can eat anything she wants and not gain an ounce," or "she never looks any older." In fact, these qualities cause suspicion after a certain age.

The qualities that endear you to others have little to do with the way you look. Your laugh, your ability to make anything an adventure, your thoughtfulness, or the purposeful way you move when you're doing what you love attracts others to you.

When you can't love and accept who you are, it is very difficult to feel love and acceptance from someone else. If you don't feel worthy or deserving of respect or adoration, you deny yourself the exquisite pleasure of being treated like royalty with the right partner.

Because so many past hurts, insults, emotions, arguments, and memories get locked in your body, opening yourself to another can be risky business. Even with partners you've known and loved for a long time, you can become self-conscious or suddenly shy, embarrassed, or otherwise unavailable. If someone has said or done something to hurt or upset you and you stuffed your emotions to avoid confrontation, you may not feel very loving towards them when they wish to get close to you.

Your body registers your emotions whether you acknowledge them or not. True intimacy begins by listening and responding to your body's wisdom. At a deep level, your body knows what's best. It is committed to protecting you at all costs. When you trust yourself, you will be able to open to others and express yourself in many creative and loving ways.

Putting it into practice

Being comfortable with your sexuality does not depend on your size, shape, age, or experience. Like charisma, when you are radiating Body Confidence, people are drawn to you because you're comfortable with yourself and delighted by those around you. You're not dwelling on what should or could have been or what might be. You are swept up in what is going on right now. Nothing could be more fascinating than what's unfolding in the moment. There's nowhere you'd rather be. And most importantly, there's no one you'd rather be than yourself.

The next time the opportunity arises, invite intimacy into your life by flirting with someone. Play peek-a-boo with a baby, tell a kid a corny joke, wink at the teller at the bank, smile at the mailman, or blow a kiss to a senior citizen. Lose yourself completely in the act of authentically connecting with another — even if it's only for a moment.

Most of us crave the intimacy that comes from touching another human being — whether it's with our hands, our hearts, or our sense of humor. But intimate moments can't occur if we're too busy criticizing others, censoring our thoughts, assuming the worst, or forbidding ourselves to feel.

Dare to share a little bit of yourself with a stranger. Dare to share a little bit of yourself with a loved one. See how this offering of intimacy opens up or closes down another. How does it make you feel?

Intimate Encounters
Exercise 10-1

Keep track of the all the ways you touch another's life by recording the incidents and accidents that bring you closer to someone. Record the following along with any unexpected outcomes.

Monday

Who was involved?_____

_____

What happened? _____

_____

_____

When did it take place?_____

Where did it take place? _____

How did it make you feel? _____

_____

Why did you connect with this person? _____

_____

Tuesday

Who was involved?_____

_____

What happened? _____

_____

_____

When did it take place? _____

Where did it take place? _____

How did it make you feel? _____

_____

Why did you connect with this person? _____

_____

Wednesday

Who was involved?_____

_____

What happened? _____

_____

_____

When did it take place?_____

Where did it take place? _____

How did it make you feel? _____

_____

Why did you connect with this person? _____

_____

Thursday

Who was involved?_____

_____

What happened? _____

_____

_____

When did it take place? _____

Where did it take place? _____

How did it make you feel? _____

_____

Why did you connect with this person? _____

_____

Friday

Who was involved?_____

_____

What happened? _____

_____

_____

When did it take place? _____

Where did it take place? _____

How did it make you feel? _____

_____

Why did you connect with this person? _____

_____

Saturday

Who was involved?_____

_____

What happened? _____

_____

_____

When did it take place? _____

Where did it take place? _____

How did it make you feel? _____

_____

Why did you connect with this person? _____

_____

Sunday

Who was involved?_____

_____

What happened? _____

_____

_____

When did it take place? _____

Where did it take place? _____

How did it make you feel? _____

_____

Why did you connect with this person? _____

_____

Lesson 29

If Body Confidence in the bedroom is about being comfortable with your private self, then Body Confidence in the boardroom is about being comfortable with your public self. How do you "power up" for an important meeting, interview, assignment, or sale? How do you present yourself? Are there certain clothes you wear, a particular way you style your hair, any rituals you perform before jumping in and facing the challenge at hand?

I used to be the membership director at an exclusive fitness resort. On the days I had appointments with potential members, I'd wear a power suit that psychologically helped me seal the deal and make a sale. When I was a club manager, I'd wear our club's polo shirts and shorts and any number of matching accessories. Other department managers would assume I was having more fun than they were simply because I was wearing casual clothes and projecting a confident, carefree attitude.

I'm not saying clothes by themselves can create confidence, but they can go a long way toward projecting a powerful or playful image. Knowing what colors, cuts, and styles make the most of your assets can go a long way towards boosting your Body Confidence. If you are serious about projecting a certain image, you may want to consider hiring an image consultant. If you've ever watched an episode of the cable television show, *What Not To Wear*, you know a person's preferences are not always in line with what they wish to project. You also know that people are pretty resistant to changing their preferences even when presented with more appropriate options.

Body Confidence in the boardroom is not just about what you're wearing. It's about how you wear it (with confidence!) and how you use your body language to back up your words, ideas, and intentions. Have you ever noticed how confident people walk, stand, sit, and communicate with others? If you haven't, start noticing how others command your attention without saying a word. Then try practicing these strategies in your life, if you are not doing so already.

Putting it into practice

The next time you head to the mall or department store, allow yourself some extra time for exploration. If you really want to have some fun, take a friend along who has no problem giving you an opinion. Then pick out a few outfits in colors or styles you wouldn't normally wear. Try them on and see how wearing them affects the way you feel about yourself.

For example, I tend to prefer turtlenecks and avoid plunging necklines or sleeveless tops. A friend recently suggested I get in touch with my "Venus" energy. She suggested I buy a couple of shirts that celebrated the feminine and flirty side of my personality. Of course I resisted at first, but eventually I conceded. I now have two or three "Venus shirts," as I like to call them, and definitely feel more flirtatious when I wear them.

Another example is the time I was helping my sister with a charity event for the American Heart Association. In the afternoon I was dressed in shorts and a polo shirt (as in my health club days). As I waited in the lobby for a luggage cart, someone asked me for directions. Apparently I looked like I worked there (probably in the health club). That evening I felt like Cinderella. Once I put on my long black gown, people who had seen me during the day didn't recognize me. Even though I was more comfortable in my shorts, an entirely different sense of Body Confidence emerged, and I embraced it.

Broadcasting Body Confidence
Exercise 10-2

1. What image are you trying to project?

   _____

2. How might that best be accomplished? _____

   _____

3. What hair style is most appropriate for the intended look?

   _____

4. What colors convey your intentions?_____

5. How does getting a manicure, pedicure, massage, facial, or great haircut make you feel?

   _____

6. What type of undergarments support (literally and figuratively) your image?

   _____

7. What posture do you assume when you intend to broadcast your power?

   _____

8. How is this different when you exude a sense of playfulness?

   _____

9. How is this different when you are feeling sexy or sassy?

   _____

10. Do you wear different scents for different occasions?_____

11. What role do accessories play in creating your intended image?

   _____

12. Have you ever consulted a professional to help you discover your style, or do you trust yourself to make the right decisions?

   _____

Lesson 30

The challenging thing about life — or is it the greatest gift? — is that just when we get used to the way it is, it changes. Even though we may have mastered Body Confidence in the bedroom and the boardroom and discovered one or the other to be more important at different times in our life, the ongoing challenge lies in creating and maintaining Body Confidence throughout our life span.

There is no doubt we live in a culture obsessed with youth and beauty. This can make anyone over a certain age feel a bit obsolete. Especially as our kids grow and don't seem to need us as much, our spouses develop new interests, or we suddenly wonder why we're wasting the best years of our lives pursuing someone else's dream.

While reading Victoria Moran's book, *Younger By the Day*, I came across a line that really rang true for me. She was describing how middle-aged women are essentially invisible in our society. Since I had been feeling invisible for what seemed like years, I was comforted to know I wasn't making this concept up.

The media tend to portray women in three stages. Beautiful, vital, sexy young women wearing the latest fashions — or not much of anything — while engaging in outrageous adventures with gorgeous guys are represented the most.

The mature woman is usually portrayed as a helpless elder taking medications for arthritis, depression, high blood pressure, high cholesterol, or any number of ailments comes in second.

The middle-aged woman, if she is represented, is either cleaning up after her family, in a quandary about what to cook for them, or playing out some version of a desperate housewife. Seldom is she seen as the sophisticated, smart, sexy, talented woman she has become.

How do we not succumb to the less than favorable role society has allocated to aging women? I propose we age gracefully. This is not to be confused with "quietly" or "invisibly." I propose we use our considerable power and voice to make a difference at home, at work, and in the world at large. From political candidates attempting to win the "women's vote" to television networks devoting entire channels to women viewers to the rise of "chick lit," women are at last being recognized as the powerful economic and political force we are.

What does Body Confidence have to do with any of this? Everything! When you feel confident enough to make the changes you desire in your own life, that confidence carries over to the world at large.

Of course, by now you know this. You are experiencing the advantages of Body Confidence and are exploring the new frontiers opening to you. I look forward to hearing about your adventures.

Putting it into practice

If you are inclined and have the time or access to a local community college or university, you may want to take a course or two in Women's Studies and Women's Health. This is a great way to learn not only about the contribution of women throughout history but also to understand the lifecycle and stages specific to women.

So much of our history, medical studies, and research have been based on the male model. Fortunately, this is changing and more research has been undertaken with the female perspective in mind. As a result, much wisdom in regards to women's health has emerged. I have listed some of my favorite authors on women's health/holistic health and their books in Resource Central.

As a final exercise, I'd like to tap into the wisdom you've gained as a result of reading and participating in this process.

Note To Self
Exercise 10-3

Is your journal full of insights, awareness of your progress, attitude adjustments, or shifts in perspective? I imagine so. If not, it's never too late to start.

Remember the first few weeks when I asked you to go for a walk or move around a bit and then settle into your body for a little soul searching? I'd like you to start off this exercise the same way. The difference is now you have lots of options. You can choose a walk, stretching, a strength training routine, or any number of activities.

Once you've returned from your workout, find a quiet corner where you'll have time to yourself to draft a very important letter. If you have some nice stationery, please use it.

Write down a series of statements about yourself that support the work you've been doing. Please write at least one full page of positive thoughts, reminders, quotes, whatever — as long as the words acknowledge and honor you at some level. Recall in detail your successes as well as the ways you are tempted to sabotage yourself and what you need to do to move beyond the setbacks. If you have a hard time doing this for yourself, imagine you are writing to letter to someone you love deeply in an effort to encourage and uplift this person.

Once you have completed this, seal it in an envelope, address it to yourself, and put it in a place where no one else will find it (but you won't forget it). When you need some support, take out your note and read it. Encouraging words at the right time can change a life. I hope the words in this book may be a few of them.

Resource Central

Introduction

Books

Mind Walks: One Hundred Easy Ways to Relieve Stress, Stay Motivated and Nourish Your Soul; Mary H. Frakes; Life Lessons (June 21, 1999)

The Spirited Walker: Fitness Walking For Clarity, Balance, and Spiritual Connection; Carolyn Scott Kortge; HarperSanFrancisco; 1st edition (May 1, 1998)

Step counters

There are as many options for step counters these days as there are budgets. These two sources are my favorites, but I encourage you to explore all the options to find the one that is right for your program.

Walk4Life; http://www.walk4life.com; 1-888-422-1806; 12137 Rhea Drive, Unit B; Plainfield, Illinois 60585

Accusplit; http://www.accusplit.com; For sales in the United States and Canada call: 800-935-1996; fax: 408-432-0316; International calls: 408-432-8228, ext.4; Email: Sales@ACCUSPLIT.com

http://walking.about.com; This website is full of information on walking programs and products.

Audiotapes and CDs

Health Journeys — Resources for the Mind, Body and Spirit; http://www.healthjourneys.com

Belleruth Naparstek has some outstanding guided visualization tapes and cds. I especially recommend her *Weight Loss* guided visualization for this group. Whether the goal is to lose weight or not, the words and affirmations are nourishing for the spirit. You can become a distributor and get CDs and tapes at a discount price. This is great for facilitating a group.

Chapter One

Books

Daily Meditation for Dieters; Ann Colby; Citadel Press (November 1, 1994)

Discovering the Body's Wisdom; Mirka Knaster; Bantam (June 1, 1996)

Nourishing Wisdom; Marc David; Harmony/Bell Tower; Reprint edition (February 15, 1994)

The Zen of Eating; Ronna Kabatznick, PhD; Perigee Trade; 1st edition (March 1, 1998)

Your Life is Your Message: Finding Harmony With Yourself, Others, and the Earth; Eknath Easwaran; Hyperion; (September 1, 1997)

Video

Master Your Metabolism — A Complete Guide to Weight Management; www.lifetimefitness.com; 1-888-430-LIFE

If you want the inside story on how your body uses the food you eat to fuel your activities, this video illustrates it well. It takes the mystery out of metabolism and gives you practical advice on how to raise your metabolism, maximize your fitness results, eat stress-free, and begin to make lifestyle changes.

Chapter Two

Books

Fit From Within: 101 Simple Secrets to Change Your Body and Your Life; Starting Today and Lasting Forever; Victoria Moran; McGraw-Hill; 1 edition (April 17, 2003)

Making Peace With Food; Susan Kano; Harper Paperbacks; Revised edition (March 1, 1989)

Cards

Medicine Cards: The Discovery of Power Through the Ways of Animals; Jamie Sams; St. Martin's Press (July 30, 1999)

Sacred Path Cards: The Discovery of Self Through Native Teachings; Jamie Sams; HarperSanFrancisco (October 12, 1990)

Websites

www.drweil.com; Many of you are familiar with Dr. Andrew Weil. His site is full of helpful information on alternative health care practices and products.

www.healthy.net; Another resource for almost any type of health-care question or concern.

www.prevention.com; You may be familiar with or subscribe to *Prevention* magazine or enjoy some of their other publications.

www.mayohealth.org -This site gives you more of the Western medical model approach to health and well-being.

Chapter Three

Audiotapes

Energy Anatomy: The Science of Personal Power, Spirituality, and Health; Carolyn Myss; Sounds True (July 1, 1997)

Creating Total Health; Christiane Northrup,MD; Sounds True (February 1, 1995)

Books

Simply Relax: An Illustrated Guide to Slowing Down and Enjoying Life; Dr. Sarah Brewer; Ulysses Press (April 1, 2000)

Why is Everyone So Cranky?: The Ten Trends Complicating Our Lives and What We Can Do About Them; C. Leslie Charles; Hyperion (October 13, 1999)

Websites

These descriptions are taken from the websites.

www.myss.com; Caroline Myss develops educational programs in human consciousness, spirituality and mysticism, health, energy medicine, and the science of medical intuition. She offers two programs, running three courses per year, on Sacred Contracts and Mysticism.

www.drnorthrup.com; Christiane Northrup, MD, obstetrician/gynecologist, is an empowering, internationally known visionary in women's health and wellness. As a practicing physician for over twenty years, Dr. Northrup is a leading proponent of medicine and healing that acknowledge the unity of the mind and body, as well as the powerful role of the human spirit in creating health.

Chapter Four

Books

Do What You Are: Discover the Perfect Career for You Through the Secrets of Personality Type; Paul D. Tieger, Barbara Barron-Tieger; Little, Brown; 3rd edition (April 1, 2001)

How You Do Anything Is How You Do Everything: A Workbook; Cheri Huber; Keep-It-Simple (June 28, 1988)

*Embracing Uncertainty: Breakthrough Methods for Achieving Peace of Mind When Facing the Unknow*n; Susan Jeffers; St. Martin's Press; 1st U.S. edition (March 10, 2003)

Websites

www.keepitsimplebooks.com; This is the website for the Center for the Practice of Zen Buddhist Meditation where you can find information on American Zen teacher Cheri Huber and the Keep It Simple Books. You can get all of her books on this site, including the *How You Do Anything is How You Do Everything* workbook and my latest favorite, *Suffering is Optional.*

http://www.truecolors.org; I was trained in this personality profile model and use it often in my seminars. It's easy to understand and apply. There are several different personality type models and many of them revolve around the same general types or categories. Having a basic understanding of personality preferences is helpful when working with groups.

Chapter Five

Audiotapes

Lighten Up: The Amazing Power of Grace Under Pressure; C.W. Metcalf-Nightingale Conant Corp (June 1, 1994)

Books

Creating Sacred Space With Feng Shui: Learn the Art of Space Clearing and Bring New Energy into Your Life; Karen Kingston; Broadway; 1st U.S. edition (January 6, 1997)

Learning to Fly: Reflections on Fear, Trust, and the Joy of Letting Go; Sam Keen; Broadway (September 5, 2000)

Making Peace With Food; Susan Kano; Harper Paperbacks; Revised edition (March 1, 1989)

Move Your Stuff, Change Your Life; Karen Rauch Carter; Fireside (January 6, 2000)

The Dance: Moving to the Rhythms of Your True Self; Oriah Mountain Dreamer; HarperSanFrancisco (September 1, 2001)

Websites

Here are a couple of fun websites to spark your "Fat vs. Thin" discussion and exercise.

www.adiosbarbie.com; Their motto is "a body image size for every body."

www.fatso.com; Their motto is "Fat! So? For people who don't apologize for their size."

Chapter Six

Books

Feeding the Body, Nourishing the Soul; Deborah Kesten; Conari Press (October 1, 1997)

Living Juicy — Daily Morsels for Your Creative Soul; SARK; Celestial Arts (September 1, 1994)

Office Yoga: Simple Stretches for Busy People; Darrin Zeer; Chronicle Books (April 1, 2000)

Stretching Lessons — The Daring That Starts Within; Sue Bender; HarperSanFrancisco; 1st edition (April, 2002)

The Art of the Moment: Simple Ways to Get the Most from Life; Veronique Vienne; Clarkson Potter; 1st edition (October 15, 2002)

The Woman's Comfort Book: A Self Nurturing Guide for Restoring Balance in Your Life; Jennifer Louden; HarperSanFrancisco; 1st edition (March 27, 1992)

Websites

www.onespirit.com; This is book club offers a variety of books, products, and other resources for the spirit, mind and body.

Chapter Seven

Books

American Heart Association Meals in Minutes; The American Heart Association; Clarkson Potter; Spiral edition (May 9, 2000)

Food & Mood; Elizabeth Somer, M.A., R.D.; Owl Books; 2nd edition (December 15, 1999)

Nutrition For Dummies; Carol Ann Rinzler; For Dummies; 2nd edition (July 1, 1999)

The American Dietetic Association's Complete Food & Nutrition Guide; Roberta Larson Duyff; Wiley; 2nd edition (August 9, 2002)

Your Body Knows Best; Anne Louise Gittleman, MS; Pocket (February 1, 1997)

Websites

www.annlouise.com; Ann Louise Gittleman, Ph.D., C.N.S., is a well respected health pioneer and nutritionist.

http://navigator.tufts.edu; This site offers a listing of the best resources on the web regarding nutrition.

http://www.nal.usda.gov/fnic/index.html; The Food and Nutrition Information Center (FNIC) at the National Agricultural Library (NAL) FNIC's website provides a directory to credible, accurate resources.

www.mypyramid.gov; Everything you need to know about the new food pyramid.

www.pueblo.gsa.gov; This site offers all kinds of valuable information from the US government.

http://therespectedwoman.com/; This is Body Confidence alumni Linda Brakeall's website. She contributed the Food Planning Guide and has much other wisdom to offer.

Chapter Eight

Books

A Woman's Book of Strength; Karen Andes; Perigee Trade; 1st edition (January 1, 1995)

The Magic of Conflict: Turning a Life of Work into a Work of Art; Thomas Crum; Touchstone (February 1, 1998)

The Art of Doing Nothing: Simple Ways to Make Time for Yourself; Veronique Vienne, Erica Lennard; Clarkson Potter; 1st edition (August 25, 1998)

The Seven Whispers; Christina Baldwin; New World Library (February 9, 2002)

The Unofficial Guide to Beating Stress; Pat Goudey Wiley; 1st edition (June 1, 2000)

Websites

www.stressedforsuccess.com; This is my website. Sign up for my for my free ezine, *Stress Less Living*, and receive tension-tackling techniques delivered to your inbox once a month.

Chapter Nine

Books

How Much Joy Can You Stand? How to Push Past Your Fears and Create Your Dreams; Suzanne Falter-Barns; Beyond Words Publishing Company (March 1, 1999)

The Bach Flower Remedies; Edward Bach, E.J. Wheeler; McGraw-Hill; 1st edition (October 11, 1998)

Energy Medicine; Donna Eden; Putnam Publishing Group (January 1, 2000)

You Can Heal Your Life; Louise L. Hay; Hay House; Gift edition (September, 1999)

Ophelia Speaks: Adolescent Girls Write About Their Search for Self; Sara Shandler; Harper Paperbacks; 1st edition (June 1, 1999)

Cards

Flower Messages; Melanie Eclare; Quadrille; (September 1, 2004)

Sacred Contracts: The Journey: an Interactive Experience for Guidance; Caroline Myss, Peter Occhiogrosso; Hay House; Package edition (March 1, 2004)

Websites

These are just a few websites that offer a wealth of information on eating disorders and can direct you to additional resources.

http://www.nationaleatingdisorders.org

http://www.something-fishy.org

http://www.caringonline.com

Chapter Ten

Books

The Comfort Queen's Guide to Life: Create All That You Need with Just What You've Got; Jennifer Louden; Harmony (May 16, 2000)

Finding Your Own North Star: Claiming the Life You Were Meant to Live; Martha Beck; Three Rivers Press; (January 29, 2002)

The Call: Discovering Why You Are Here; Oriah Mountain Dreamer; HarperSanFrancisco (September 1, 2003)

The Intuitive Way: A Guide to Living from Inner Wisdom; Penney Peirce; Beyond Words Publishing (September 1, 1997)

The Invitation; Oriah Mountain Dreamer; Harpercollins; 1st edition (February, 1999)

I Will Not Die an Unlived Life: Reclaiming Purpose and Passion; Dawna Markova; Conari Press (October 15, 2000)

The Art of Growing Up: Simple Ways to Be Yourself at Last; Veronique Vienne, Jeanne Lipsey; Clarkson Potter; 1st edition (October 10, 2000)

Women's Bodies, Women's Wisdom; Christiane Northrup; Bantam (March, 1998)

Younger by the Day: 365 Ways to Rejuvenate Your Body and Revitalize Your Spirit; Victoria Moran; HarperSanFrancisco (December 1, 2004)

Websites

www.body-confidence.com — This is where your journey begins. Join the online community and continue to receive the support you need the develop and maintain Body Confidence.

Facilitating Body Confidence

Leading a Body Confidence Group

This part of the book is for those of you who would like to start a Body Confidence program in your community, school, church, neighborhood, work environment, or just with a couple of girlfriends. What follows are basic suggestions and guidelines for you to follow.

In Eight Essentials for Facilitators I've listed the qualities, questions, and concepts you need to consider before starting a group. In the Planning Pages section, I've listed the items you'll want to have on hand each week, the learning objectives for each chapter, discussion topics, handouts, and homework along with a sample agenda.

I have not included marketing materials such as flyers or press releases or sample ads. How you run your program is up to you. I don't want to limit your creativity. I do suggest you give yourself enough time to adequately plan and promote the program. For me, six to eight weeks is the minimum planning time. You may need to offer free introductory classes and talk to various groups to generate some excitement. Set a realistic target date you are committed to keeping and then do at least one thing every day to organize the details and promote the program.

You can also consult the website www.body-confidence.com and email me directly if you have questions or suggestions or need a last minute pep talk. Now, take a deep breath and let the games begin!

Eight Essentials for Facilitators

Okay, so you've worked through the program and are familiar with the exercises, philosophies, and principles of Body Confidence. Now you are ready to share this information with others.

Many of you may be teachers, trainers, coaches, or therapists who have ample experience facilitating. In that case, you may already have a sense of how you would like to adapt and organize the material for your particular group. However, if this is your first time facilitating, I will walk you through what I consider the Eight Essentials for Facilitators:

1. Know your audience
2. Know yourself
3. Let your personality shine
4. Have a plan
5. Expect the unexpected
6. Model what you expect
7. Trust the process
8. Enjoy the process

After you have facilitated the program a time or two you will know what works best. In the beginning, if you stick with these basics, you will be off to an excellent start.

1. Know your audience

Just as you started the Body Confidence program with a series of questions – who, what, when, where, why, and how —begin to get a sense of your group by playing twenty questions. If you don't know the answers, ask! Call people you think would be perfect participants and get their feedback. If you can't think of anyone, tap into whatever communities you currently have access to and ask their opinions.

1. Who is my audience?
2. How do they spend their time?

3. Where do they live?

4. How old are they?

5. What do they value?

6. Why would this be important to them?

7. How will I market to them?

8. What would make this worth their time, money, and energy?

9. What needs do they have that are not being met?

10. How much money do they make?

11. How much would they be willing to pay for the program?

12. How far would they be willing to travel?

13. When is the most convenient time for them to attend?

14. How can I reduce the risk for the participant?

15. What guarantees might they need?

16. What incentives would encourage people to take immediate action?

17. What kind of discounts could I offer to friends who sign up together as Body Confidence Buddies?

18. When is the best time of year to start this program?

19. What would make this program a success for them?

20. What follow up services or programs might they want?

Although you can adapt this material to teens and younger children, many of you will be working with adults. Understanding the foundation of adult learning theories will help you capture your participants' interest quickly and communicate with them effectively throughout the workshop. The following are a few basic concepts of adult learning theories.

- Adult learners must feel "safe" in the learning environment.

  Before participants will communicate what is important to them, they must be able to trust that what they share will be respected.

Make sure each participant acknowledges the request for confidentiality. Help lower participants' anxiety by reinforcing that their experience will be interesting and worthwhile. Invite participants to learn by modeling, experimenting, observing, and interacting with others. Positive feedback is essential.

- The richest resources for learning reside in learners themselves.

  As anxious as you may be to share your knowledge with them, participants will learn just as much from each other as they will from you. Your job is to introduce the topic and facilitate the discussion. Let them talk. The traditional teacher/student relationship does not work effectively in this setting. Value their experience.

- Adults insist that new learning is personally relevant and useful.

  Give participants time to reflect on what is being presented and relate it to their own lives. Make extracurricular activities part of the program. Use a number of resources for learning — music, movies, magazines, newspaper articles, etc.

- Adults learn best in small chunks of information.

  Present the topic in small chunks through a variety of sensory modes. Repeating the information three times during a session in different ways aids in retention and allows patterns of learning to emerge.

- Clearly define learning objectives or outcomes for adult learners.

  Adult learners want to know why they need to know certain skills or information. Ask them what they want out of this course. Let them establish their personal learning objectives and goals. You may guide them or make suggestions, but encourage them to be their own expert.

2. Know yourself

You may have heard the expression, "If you don't know where you're going, any road will take you there." To be an effective leader and inspire others to follow a similar path, you must know where you're going and why, what route you're taking, what you'll need along the way, and when you expect to arrive. There will undoubtedly be "construction" along the way, but you must start out with your destination in mind.

I must admit the first Body Confidence email course started out with no specific destination in mind. I knew what direction I was heading, but the path itself was not clearly marked. It wasn't until I made the journey a time or two that I gained enough confidence to map it out for others.

Even though you now hold that map in your hands, there are still certain questions only you can answer. Here are a few of them.

1. What do I hope to gain from facilitating this program?
2. What wisdom do I hope to impart to others?
3. How does it support my other goals?
4. What unique gifts, talents, or experiences do I bring to the topic?
5. How much energy do I have to devote to making this a success?
6. When is the best time for me to offer this program?
7. How much time do I have to market and promote the program?
8. Who do I know who can help me during the various stages of the program?
9. What resources do I have that I can use for the program?
10. What facilities do I have access to that offer meeting rooms, workout spaces, walking trails, kitchens, or other resources I might need?
11. How committed am I to creating a new community?
12. What complementary businesses or resources can I collaborate with to market and promote the program?
13. What would I consider a wildly successful outcome for my first workshop?
14. What other services or products might I offer to follow up with this program?

15. How willing am I to get additional training?

3. Let your personality shine

If you are not inspired, your ability to inspire others will be greatly diminished. Most of you are not stand-up comedians or top billing on the motivational speaker circuit, but all of you have unique personalities. Just ask anyone who loves you.

The best facilitators are not those who pretend to be the world's leading expert in their field. (While that can be impressive, often times it's just annoying.) The best facilitators are those who can be themselves. They tap into their unique blend of wisdom, experience, and intuition and share it with the group.

I have a certain way of writing and presenting that may be very different from your way. While my essays and ideas will guide the group, you will lead them. You will be the community leader and the reason people show up.

Don't be afraid to be yourself. The world needs more originals.

4. Have a plan

If you decide to follow the twelve-week plan outlined in this book, then this step will be relatively easy for you. In the next section, I've provided planning pages and possible agendas. If, however, you have more or less time to deliver the program, then you'll need to do some creative planning.

Also, because not all who read this book will become a part of a group, the exercises are designed for individuals to do on their own. However, in a group setting, the emphasis needs to be on group activities so that participants have plenty of opportunities to learn from each other. Find ways for participants to share their experiences and insights with the exercises in small groups or with a BC Buddy.

It's my experience that it's better to have too much material and too many options than not enough. You will also want to have a couple of different ways to illustrate the same point. Use your answers from the questions in "Know Yourself" to help you plan your agenda.

We all have preferred methods of learning new material, so make sure that you accommodate as many different learning styles as possible. If you are not familiar with your own personality preferences and your dominant ways of learning, I encourage you to find out. It's important that you not only know your preferred style but also are aware of other styles so you can learn how to effectively relate to them.

You will also do best to stick to your plan unless the plan is definitely not working. As a facilitator, it is easy to jump to the conclusion that your ideas are bombing when, in fact, it may just be taking awhile for participants to understand the concepts and act on them. Remember, you have worked with the material a lot longer than they have.

Try presenting the same concept in a couple of different ways. Give plenty of examples and options. Don't assume you are wrong if you don't get it right the first time. With time and experience you'll learn when to deviate from the plan and add something more appropriate or relevant to your group.

5. Expect the unexpected

One thing you can't plan for but can expect is the unexpected. "Unexpected," by its very definition, means without advance planning or warning. Instead of imagining the worst case scenario and assuming all unexpected events are unwelcome, let me assure you that whatever happens, you will be able to work with it.

Many times the most memorable things that happen in workshops are things I couldn't have planned or imagined. Insights are often sparked by a story someone casually mentions or an action someone spontaneously takes or a song, movie, or poem that comes to mind during a discussion.

I believe when our intentions, thoughts, and actions are aligned, anything can happen. When you put a group of equally aligned individuals in one area, certainly something is bound to happen.

Of course the occasional mishap, miscommunication, or mismanagement can trip you up from time to time. Consider it a test of your creativity and resiliency, not to mention stress management skills, to overcome adversity.

As much as you may prefer perfection, you can live with excellence. Excellence is almost always good enough. If you're committed to excellence, I'm convinced things will work out for the best — no matter what you get to work with.

6. Model what you expect

The "do what I say, not what I do" method of teaching is not my idea of excellence. If you want your participants to be on time, you need to be on time. If you want your participants to be prepared, you must be prepared. If you want them to exude Body Confidence, you have to exude Body Confidence.

This doesn't mean that you're always on guard and can never make a mistake. You're human and things happen. It's just if you want to be a credible resource to others, you have to embody the principles you are promoting.

I often tell my students I won't make them do anything I won't do as well. This helps them relax and trust they are going to be safe. It also reminds them we're in this together.

You can't expect others to do what you are not willing to do. Give your participants every reason to relax and trust you.

7. Trust the process

In order for participants to trust you, you must first trust the process. In my corporate training experience, I've learned that no matter how things appear, if you have a plan, pay attention to the people, and trust your-self to do and say what is needed, you will do well. And you will learn as much as you teach.

You can teach the same material to seven different groups and have seven different experiences. You can say the same words in the same way and get a totally different response.

What you have to remember when you're not getting the response you want is that you are meeting people where they are, not where you'd like them to be. Some people may not be ready to hear your message at this point in their lives. Don't assume there is something wrong with you or the material.

I know Body Confidence can change lives. I've witnessed it over and over again. I've also witnessed people return to familiar patterns and predictable routines that prevent them from reaching their goals, con-vinced it was the program that didn't work, not them.

You can not change anyone else. You can only be a catalyst for change. Not everyone is on your time schedule.

The ones who are ready will amaze you with their courage, delight you with their determination, and love you for being the one to light the way. What could be more rewarding than that?

8. Enjoy the process

Putting a program together and facilitating a group will require a lot from you. It will also require a lot from your participants. It may take awhile before you get results. At some point in the process you may regret spending your time, energy, and money.

There. Now you know. I'm telling you up front. I don't want you to think this is easy. It isn't. But it will lead you to some pretty heady places.

You will find out what an incredible leader you are. You will discover how much your wisdom matters. You will know how exciting it is to be a positive resource for others. You will experience the thrill of assisting others in reaching their goals.

You will increase your strength, flexibility, and endurance as you put yourself through the paces. It will be a challenge. It will also be immensely rewarding. Savor the small successes. Connect deeply with your participants. Dare to open your heart as well as your mind.

One of the best gifts you can offer others is your love of life. Be generous with your joy.

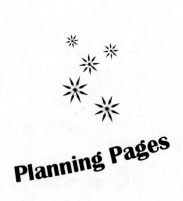

Planning Pages

Introductory Session

Items to Have on Hand

- Name tags
- 3 x 5 cards
- 3-ring binders for Body Confidence Journal pages
- Step counters (if you are providing them as part of program)
- Guided visualization tapes or CDs
- Portable stereo for playing music for energy breaks and meditation
- Candle and matches for meditation/visualization (optional/depending on safety codes)
- Extra pens or pencils
- White board, easel with writing pads, poster boards, markers

Other Resources

Equipment: _____

Music:_____

Resources: Books/Articles/Videos: _____

_____

Quotes, Poems, Pictures: _____

_____

Preparation Time:

- Familiarize yourself with the material. Make copies of handouts.
- Select music for energy breaks and closing.
- Select and rehearse visualization or guided meditation script.
- Set up the room, creating an inviting environment.

Calculating Your Class Time:

- 25–30% on introductions, agendas, expectations — it is essential to get the off on the right foot, feeling comfortable, knowing what to expect, and anticipating future classes
- 25–30% discussion/lecture
- 40–50% experiential learning through handouts, activities,

movement, meditation

- There are usually more handouts than there is time to do them. Don't worry if you don't get a chance to introduce them all. It's more important that participants experience the group activities and participate in feedback and discussion. A large part of the learning comes from this interaction. You can always assign the handouts as homework and discuss them during the next session's check-in/feedback segment.

Learning Objectives:

- Agree on group guidelines.
- Introduce overview of course.
- Explain how to use BC Journal pages and the importance of keeping track of progress.
- Read through and sign the Awareness Agreement on page 163.
- Make sure you have the correct contact information on individuals and agree on how participants can connect with each other in between classes. (You can use 3 x 5 cards to have participants write down their contact information and note whether they want it shared with the group. Then you can distribute a list of everyone's information at the next meeting.)
- Introduce the concept of a Body Confidence project, such as a collage, video, or audio tape depicting Body Confidence, to be shared at the final meeting.

Discussion Topics:

- What makes a group successful?
- What standards are you willing to commit to for the duration of the course?
- What drew you to this program at this time?
- What's your vision for yourself?

Experiential Exercise

- Present a mix-and-mingle or icebreaker type of exercise that gets participants talking and sharing ideas with each other. (Whole Person Associates publishes books for facilitators that are filled with games trainers can play with groups.)
- If you include step counters as part of your program, use this time for participants to set them up and practice using them.

Handouts and Exercises
- Awareness Agreement
- BC Journal pages

Homework:
- BC Journal Daily Recaps

Introductory Session Outline

Taking Care of Business
- Introductions
- Awareness Agreement

Discussion Topics
- Course overview
- Expectations and assumptions
- Using the Body Confidence Journal
- Body Confidence project

Experiential Exercises
- Mix and mingle
- Try out step counters

Handouts
- Awareness Agreement
- Daily Recap pages

Homework
- BC Journal Daily Recaps

Closing Circle

Body Confidence from the Inside Out Awareness Agreement

1. I am participating in a program that encourages me to review my attitudes, behaviors, and choices with regard to diet, exercise, and body image.

2. I understand this is not a counseling program.

3. I agree to read the lessons and participate in the exercises.

4. I am making a commitment to live an active, healthy lifestyle on a day-to-day basis.

5. I agree to be patient and compassionate with myself as I learn to nourish my mind, body, and spirit.

6. I agree to participate in regular physical activity that includes aerobic conditioning, strength training, and flexibility exercises.

7. I agree to eat a sensible diet that provides necessary nutrients from a variety of foods.

8. I allow myself to have "good days" and "bad days" as I commit to a healthy lifestyle. Bad days do not justify giving up on myself or dropping out of the program.

9. I agree to investigate the facts and find out what works best for me in relation to eating, exercising, reducing stress, and integrating the various components of healthy lifestyle.

10. I realize the way I approach and participate in this program is my responsibility. I am responsible for my attitudes, behaviors, and choices.

11. I trust in the process and let go of unrealistic expectations and predetermined outcomes.

12. I accept myself as I am right now, regardless of my alleged imperfections.

13. If I weigh myself, I will only do so once a week at the same time each week.

14. I agree to work through my resistance, summon my courage, and commit myself to a very worthy cause — the emergence of my own Body Confidence.

15. I respect the confidentiality of the group and each participant. If I need additional help, I will seek it out.

_____   _____
Your Signature   Today's Date

Chapter One – What Happened?

Items to Have on Hand
- Name tags
- Portable stereo for playing music for energy breaks and meditation
- Deck of cards — take out Jacks, Queens, Kings, Aces; use numbers 2–10 for What Are You Broadcasting? exercise
- Candle and matches for meditation/visualization (optional/depending on safety codes)
- Extra pens or pencils
- White board, easel with writing pads, poster boards, markers

Other Resources
Equipment: _____

Music:_____

Resources: Books/Articles/Videos: _____

_____

Quotes, Poems, Pictures: _____

_____

Preparation Time:
- Familiarize yourself with the material. Make copies of handouts.
- Select music for energy breaks and closing.
- Select and rehearse visualization or guided meditation script.
- Set up the room, creating an inviting environment.

Learning Objectives:
- Find out what participants expect from program.
- Discover what events contributed to or destroyed their experience of Body Confidence.
- Ascertain what participants might do now to recover and develop Body Confidence.
- Introduce and explain how to use Daily Recap BC Journal sheets.

Discussion Topics:

- What does Body Confidence mean to you?
- What are you willing to do to develop Body Confidence?
- What's missing in your health and wellness picture?
- What's your vision for yourself?

Experiential Exercise

- What Are You Broadcasting?

  Get out a deck of cards with numbers from 2–10. Ask participants to pick a card and then walk from Point A to Point B "broadcasting" the number on the card. For example, if someone draws a 2, she may slowly meander around the room with her head down, eyes averted, and shoulders slumped. If someone draws a 10, she may look people in the eye, smile, stand tall, and walk purposefully in a specific direction. Have the other participants try to guess the "broadcaster's" number. Have as many participants do this exercise as possible so they can get an idea of what it feels like in their bodies to broadcast certain messages.

Handouts and Exercises

- Who, What, When, Where, Why, & How
- BC Quotient
- 15 Things I Love To Do

Homework:

- BC Journal Daily Recaps

Chapter One Session Outline

Taking Care of Business

- Introductions
- Expectations & Assumptions
- Collect Any Remaining Awareness Agreements

Discussion Topics

- What is Body Confidence?
- Why do you need it?
- What are you willing to do to develop it?

Experiential Exercise
- What Are You Broadcasting?

Handouts
- Who, What, When, Where, Why, and How?
- Body Confidence Quotient
- 15 Things I Love to Do

Homework
- BC Journal Daily Recaps

Closing Circle

Chapter Two — Start Where You Are

Items to Have on Hand:
- Name tags
- Portable stereo for playing music for energy breaks and meditation
- Hula hoops, jump ropes, balance balls — fun and inviting exercise equipment
- Candle and matches for meditation/visualization (optional/depending on safety codes)
- Extra pens or pencils
- White board, easel with writing pads, poster boards, markers

Other Resources

Equipment: _____

Music:_____

Resources: Books/Articles/Videos: _____

_____

Quotes, Poems, Pictures: _____

_____

Preparation Time:
- Familiarize yourself with the material. Make copies of handouts.
- Select music for energy breaks and closing.
- Select and rehearse visualization or guided meditation script.
- Set up the room, creating an inviting environment.

Learning Objectives:
- Discover participants' starting points.
- Uncover current attitudes, beliefs, choices
- Determine how they see themselves as athletes or spectators.
- Find stories — or tall tales — that support their perspective.

Discussion Topics:
- Do you suffer "delusions of slender grandeur"?
- What do you think would be possible if you were 20 pounds

lighter that is not happening now?

- What did you learn from your answers to the speed writing exercise?
- Are you an athlete or a spectator?
- What stories support this assumption?
- If you are a spectator, how might you "get in the game"?

Energy Break:

- Use hula hoops, balance balls, or jump ropes to make movement fun and inviting.

Handouts and Exercises

- Speed Writing
- Athlete or Spectator
- Progress Report

Homework:

- BC Journal Daily Recaps
- Encouraging Words

  To stay engaged with the process and connected to your goal, Eric Maisel, PhD *(Coaching the Artist Within)* suggests that you to write encouraging words on note cards and keep them near your work. For example, while writing this book, I wrote things like, "You fascinate me!" "I can't wait to see how you turn out!" "You are so intriguing!" and scattered them throughout the manuscript. That way, whenever I got overwhelmed or discouraged, I could look at the material from a different point of view. Like a baby kicking in my belly, I could be curious not just uncomfortable: "What are you kicking about today?" "How can I support you today?"

  You might offer this exercise to your participants. Or utilize it yourself!

Chapter Two Session Outline

Taking Care of Business

- Welcome/Check In
- Feedback/Progress Report

Discussion Topics
- Your current ABCs
- Delusions of slender grandeur?
- Are you an athlete or spectator?

Energy Break
- Play with the hula hoops, jump ropes, or balance balls.

Handouts
- Speed Writing
- Athlete or Spectator

Homework
- Progress Report
- BC Journal Daily Recaps
- Encouraging Words

Closing Circle

Chapter Three — Examine Your Expectations

Items to Have on Hand

- Name tags
- Portable stereo for playing music for energy breaks and meditation
- Candle and matches for meditation/visualization (optional/depending on safety codes)
- Extra pens or pencils
- White board, easel with writing pads, poster boards, markers

Other Resources

Equipment: _____

Music:_____

Resources: Books/Articles/Videos: _____

_____

Quotes, Poems, Pictures: _____

_____

Preparation Time:

- Familiarize yourself with the material. Make copies of handouts.
- Select music for energy breaks and closing.
- Select and rehearse visualization or guided meditation script.
- Set up the room, creating an inviting environment.

Learning Objectives:

- Discover how participants' expectations affect their outcomes.
- Identify support systems.
- Determine how these systems support or sabotage progress.
- Identify family of origin and current family perspectives.

Discussion Topics:

- Who is included in your circle of support?
- How will the changes you are implementing affect them?
- What unconscious expectations are sabotaging your efforts?

- What expectations did you inherit?

Energy Break
- An option for this week's energy break is to teach the group a line dance, revive an oldie like the twist, or try something sassy like salsa.

Handouts and Exercises
- Support System
- Expectations
- Family of Origin
- Current Family or Community

Homework
- BC Journal Daily Recaps

Chapter Three Session Outline

Taking Care of Business
- Welcome/Check In
- Feedback/Progress Report

Discussion Topics
- Does your environment support change?
- Circle of support
- Expectations
- Your inheritance

Energy Break
- Electric Slide
- Twist
- Salsa

Handouts
- Support System
- Expectations
- Family of Origin
- Current Family or Community

Homework
- BC Journal Daily Recaps
- Closing Circle

Chapter Four — Explore Your Options

Items to Have on Hand
- Name tags
- Portable stereo for playing music for energy breaks and meditation
- Candle and matches for meditation/visualization (optional/depending on safety codes)
- Extra pens or pencils
- White board, easel with writing pads, poster boards, markers

Other Resources

Equipment: _____

Music:_____

Resources: Books/Articles/Videos: _____

_____

Quotes, Poems, Pictures: _____

_____

Preparation Time:
- Familiarize yourself with the material. Make copies of handouts.
- Select music for energy breaks and closing.
- Select and rehearse visualization or guided meditation script.
- Set up the room, creating an inviting environment.

Learning Objectives:
- Discover predictable patterns.
- Identify empowering ways to work with patterns.
- Draw unlikely conclusions that lead to insights.
- Determine how to choose wisely and commit vs. being overwhelmed by options.

Discussion Topics:
- How do you like to prefer to do things?
- Where do these patterns show up in other areas of your life?
- How do they serve you? How do they trip you up? How can you

work with them?
- How do you manage all your options?
- When do you know which option to choose and commit to?
- What are the perils of perfectionism?

Experiential Exercise
- Yes or No?

  What does a "yes" feel like in your body? Think of something you really are excited about and committed to. How does your body feel when you think about this? What does a "no" feel like? Think about something you don't what to do. How does your body feel when you think about this? Our bodies are exceptional barometers of our emotional state. Next time you are asked a question, drop down and listen to your body before you answer.

Handouts and Exercises
- What's Your Preference
- Treasure Hunt
- The Choice Is Yours

Homework:
- BC Journal Daily Recaps

Chapter Four Session Outline

Taking Care of Business
- Welcome/Check In
- Feedback/Progress Report

Discussion Topics
- Picking up on patterns
- Where do these patterns play out in other areas?
- Choosing and committing

Experiential Exercise
- Yes or No?

Handouts

- What's Your Preference
- Treasure Hunt
- The Choice Is Yours

Homework

- BC Journal Daily Recaps

Closing Circle

Chapter Five — Lighten Your Load

Items to Have on Hand

- Name tags
- Portable stereo for playing music for energy breaks & meditation
- Clown noses, Viking hats, goofy glasses, toys for the table
- Candle and matches for meditation/visualization (optional/depending on safety codes)
- Extra pens or pencils
- White board, easel with writing pads, poster boards, markers

Other Resources

Equipment: _____

Music:_____

Resources: Books/Articles/Videos: _____

_____

Quotes, Poems, Pictures: _____

_____

Preparation Time:

- Familiarize yourself with the material. Make copies of handouts.
- Select music for energy breaks and closing.
- Select and rehearse visualization or guided meditation script.
- Set up the room, creating an inviting environment.

Learning Objectives:

- Expose participants' biases in relation to weight and worthiness.
- Identify extra baggage — physical, emotional, mental.
- Develop strategies to lighten up, let go, and laugh.

Discussion Topics:

- Are you dying to be thin?
- Cultural and personal biases about weight
- What are you holding on to that is weighing you down?
- Can clearing out your closets be the key to making room for positive change?

Energy Break
- Use toys, hats, noses to create some fun for everyone — participants can perform a skit, have an impromptu puppet show, or perform a song and dance number

Handouts and Exercises
- Fat vs. Thin
- Questions to Consider
- Closet Cleaning Tips

Homework:
- BC Journal Daily Recaps
- Clean That Closet!

Chapter Five Session Outline

Taking Care of Business
- Welcome/Check In
- Feedback/Progress Report

Discussion Topics
- Dying to be thin
- Too fat for what?
- What are you holding on to?
- Clear out the clutter

Energy Break
- Play Time!

Handouts
- Fat vs. Thin
- Questions to Consider
- Closet Cleaning Tips

Homework
- BC Journal Daily Recaps
- Closet Cleaning

Closing Circle

Chapter Six — Stretch Your Knowledge

Items to Have on Hand
- Name tags
- Portable stereo for playing music for energy breaks & meditation
- Candle and matches for meditation/visualization (optional/depending on safety codes)
- Extra pens or pencils
- White board, easel with writing pads, poster boards, markers

Other Resources

Equipment: _____

Music:_____

Resources: Books/Articles/Videos: _____

_____

Quotes, Poems, Pictures: _____

_____

Preparation Time:
- Familiarize yourself with the material. Make copies of handouts.
- Select music for energy breaks and closing.
- Select and rehearse visualization or guided meditation script.
- Set up the room, creating an inviting environment.
- Learn a line dance or another easy-to-teach dance to share with the group.

Learning Objectives:
- Discover how participants' expectations affect their outcomes.
- Identify support systems.
- Determine how these systems support or sabotage progress.
- Identify family of origin and current family perspectives.

Discussion Topics:
- Who is included in your circle of support?
- How will the changes you are implementing affect them?

- What unconscious expectations are sabotaging your efforts?
- What expectations did you inherit?

Energy Break
- An option for this week's energy break is to teach the group a line dance, revive an oldie like the twist, or try something sassy like salsa.

Handouts and Exercises
- Support System
- Expectations
- Family of Origin
- Current Family or Community

Homework:
- BC Journal Daily Recaps

Chapter Six Session Outline

Taking Care of Business
- Welcome/Check In
- Feedback/Progress Report

Discussion Topics
- Does your environment support change?
- Circle of support
- Expectations
- Your inheritance

Energy Break
- Electric Slide
- Twist
- Salsa

Handouts
- Support System
- Expectations
- Family of Origin

- Current Family or Community

Homework
- BC Journal Daily Recaps
- Encouraging Words

Closing Circle

Chapter Seven — Feed Your Curiosity

Items to Have on Hand

- Name tags
- Portable stereo for playing music for energy breaks & meditation
- Candle and matches for meditation/visualization (optional/depending on safety codes)
- Extra pens or pencils
- White board, easel with writing pads, poster boards, markers
- Different types of foods with food labels on the packaging

Other Resources

Equipment: _____

Music:_____

Resources: Books/Articles/Videos: _____

_____

Quotes, Poems, Pictures: _____

_____

Preparation Time:

- Familiarize yourself with the material. Make copies of handouts.
- Select music for energy breaks and closing.
- Select and rehearse visualization or guided meditation script.
- Set up the room, creating an inviting environment.
- An option for this week's experiential exercise is to bring common food products in to help interpret labels or actually plan a field trip to the grocery store to read labels and help make nutritious food choices.

Learning Objectives:

- Cover nutrition basics.
- Identify food pyramids and other dietary guidelines.
- Interpret food labels.
- Discover how advertising affects your choices and how to spot misleading terms.

Discussion Topics:
- Basics of nutrition
- Food pyramids — cultural differences
- What nourishes you — what foods, what environment, what relationships?
- What influences your food choices?
- What makes for a great meal?
- How do you interpret food labels?

Experiential Exercise
- Bring in various foods and read labels or make a poster of a food label and define terms or take a trip to the supermarket and check out labels, marketing terms, advertising ideas, and product placement. Notice how all of these thing influence your purchasing decisions.

Handouts and Exercises
- The Last Supper
- The Foods You Choose
- Food Planning Guide

Homework:
- BC Journal Daily Recaps

Chapter Seven Session Outline

Taking Care of Business
- Welcome/Check In
- Feedback/Progress Report

Discussion Topics
- Nutrition 101
- Food pyramids
- What nourishes you: food, environment, relationships?
- What Influences your food choices?
- What makes a great meal?

Experiential Exercise
- Read Your Food Labels
- Trip to the Grocery Store

Handouts
- The Last Supper
- The Foods You Choose
- Food Planning Guide

Homework
- BC Journal Daily Recaps

Closing Circle

Chapter Eight — Build Your Personal Power

Items To Have On Hand
- Name tags
- Portable stereo for playing music for energy breaks & meditation
- Candle and matches for meditation/visualization (optional/depending on safety codes)
- Extra pens or pencils
- White board, easel with writing pads, poster boards, markers

Other Resources

Equipment: _____

Music:_____

Resources: Books/Articles/Videos: _____

_____

Quotes, Poems, Pictures: _____

_____

Preparation Time:
- Familiarize yourself with the material. Make copies of handouts.
- Select music for energy breaks and closing.
- Select and rehearse visualization or guided meditation script.
- Set up the room, creating an inviting environment.

Learning Objectives:
- Discover the impact of stress on participants' heath
- Identify where stress shows up in the body
- Identify reactions to stress: fight, flee, freeze, flow
- Outline strategies for reducing stress
- List benefits of becoming strong and working with resistance

Discussion Topics:
- How does stress affect you?
- How do you respond to stress — fight, flee, freeze, or flow?

- What ways can you combat stress?
- What are some benefits to becoming strong?

Energy Break
- Breathing Basics — take the group through a series of deep breathing exercises
- Relaxation Visualization — follow the script to lead participants through relaxation visualization

Handouts & Exercises to Illustrate:
- All Stressed Out
- I Feel It Here
- Stress Detector
- Becoming Strong

Homework:
- BC Journal Daily Recaps

Chapter Eight Session Outline

Taking Care of Business
- Welcome/Check In
- Feedback/Progress Report

Discussion Topics
- How does stress affect you?
- Fight, flight, freeze, flow
- Stress reducing strategies
- What are the benefits of being strong?

Energy Break
- Breathing Basics
- Relaxation Visualization

Handouts
- All Stressed Out
- I Feel It Here
- Stress Detector

- Becoming Strong

Homework

- BC Journal Daily Recaps

Closing Circle

Chapter Nine — Move Into Your Life

Items to Have on Hand

- Name tags
- Different styles of music for Energy Break or various instruments
- Portable stereo for playing music for energy breaks & meditation
- Candle and matches for meditation/visualization (optional/depending on safety codes)
- Extra pens or pencils
- White board, easel with writing pads, poster boards, markers

Other Resources

Equipment: _____

Music:_____

Resources: Books/Articles/Videos: _____

_____

Quotes, Poems, Pictures: _____

_____

Preparation Time:

- Familiarize yourself with the material. Make copies of handouts.
- Select music for energy breaks and closing.
- Select and rehearse visualization or guided meditation script.
- Set up the room, creating an inviting environment.

Learning Objectives:

- Identify individual rhythms — how do participants move through their day?
- Become aware of the power of music, silence, movement, and stillness.
- Identify predominant archetypes and how they show up in people's lives and bodies.
- Identify components of fitness.
- Create a personal definition of Body Confidence.

Discussion Topics:
- How do you move through your day?
- How important is music in your life?
- How would you describe your "look"?
- What kind of flower are you?
- What do you need to blossom?
- What is your personal definition of Body Confidence? How does it all fit together?

Energy Break
- Experiment with different ways to move to different types of music. A game like musical chairs may be fun to play – something that playfully makes participants aware of how music moves and motivates them

Handouts and Exercises
- I've Got the Music In Me
- Are You My Archetype
- Venn Diagrams

Homework:
- BC Journal Daily Recaps

Chapter Nine Session Outline

Taking Care of Business
- Welcome/Check In
- Feedback/Progress Report

Discussion Topics
- What moves you?
- What is your theme song?
- How do you move?
- What archetype are you?
- What kind of flower are you? What do you need to blossom?

Energy Break
- Musical Chairs

Handouts
- I've Got The Music In Me
- Are You My Archetype
- Venn Diagrams

Homework
- BC Journal Daily Recaps

Closing Circle

Chapter Ten — Body Confidence in the Bedroom, Boardroom & Beyond

Items to Have on Hand
- Name tags
- Portable stereo for playing music for energy breaks and meditation
- Candle and matches for meditation/visualization (optional/depending on safety codes)
- Extra pens or pencils
- White board, easel with writing pads, poster boards, markers
- Magazines and other materials for the collage

Other Resources

Equipment: _____

Music:_____

Resources: Books/Articles/Videos: _____

_____

Quotes, Poems, Pictures: _____

_____

Preparation Time:
- Familiarize yourself with the material. Make copies of handouts.
- Select music for energy breaks and closing.
- Select and rehearse visualization or guided meditation script.
- Set up the room, creating an inviting environment.

Learning Objectives:
- Discover how media represent women at different ages.
- Discuss elements of intimacy.
- Become aware of how clothes create an image or style.
- Share ideas on aging gracefully.
- Understand women's economic influence.

Discussion Topics:

- Who radiates Body Confidence?
- How do the media represent women?
- How is that changing as women become a powerful economic force?
- Body Confidence in the bedroom
- Body Confidence in the boardroom
- Ideas on aging gracefully
- How do clothes affect your self-image?

Experiential Exercise

- Body Confidence collage

Handouts and Exercises

- Intimate Encounters
- Broadcasting Body Confidence
- Note to Self

Homework:

- BC Journal Daily Recaps

Chapter Ten Session Outline

Taking Care of Business

- Welcome/Check In
- Feedback/Progress Report

Discussion Topics

- Who exudes body confidence?
- What role does Body Confidence play in the bedroom?
- What role does Body Confidence play in the boardroom?
- How do the media define women?

Experiential Exercise

- Body Confidence collage

Handouts

- Intimate Encounters
- Broadcasting Body Confidence
- Note to Self

Homework

- BC Journal Daily Recaps
- Encouraging Words
- Complete Body Confidence projects in preparation for sharing during the final session

Closing Circle

Closing Session

Items to Have on Hand

- Name tags
- Graduation certificates
- Portable stereo for playing music for energy breaks and meditation
- Candle and matches for meditation/visualization (optional/depending on safety codes)
- Extra pens or pencils
- White board, easel with writing pads, poster boards, markers

Other Resources

Equipment: _____

Music:_____

Resources: Books/Articles/Videos: _____

_____

Quotes, Poems, Pictures: _____

_____

Preparation Time:

- Familiarize yourself with the material. Make copies of handouts.
- Select music for energy breaks and closing.
- Select and rehearse visualization or guided meditation script.
- Set up the room, creating an inviting environment.
- Prepare graduation certificates.

Learning Objectives:

- Celebrate each individual's progress.
- Understand each ending is a new beginning.
- Learn maintenance strategies to support continued success.

Discussion Topics:

- Are your support systems in place?
- What are some strategies to help you maintain your success?

- What were the key lessons you learned from this workshop?

Experiential Exercise

- Body Confidence Project (as introduced in the first session): This project provides participants with a chance to illustrate what Body Confidence means to them. They can collect pictures of people who exude Body Confidence and paste them on poster board. Or they may want to select video clips or music or develop any creative project that expresses their vision and helps them achieve it

Handouts and Exercises

- Intimate Encounters
- Broadcasting Body Confidence
- Note to Self

Homework:

- BC Journal Daily Recaps

Closing Session Outline

Taking Care of Business

- Welcome/Check In
- Feedback/Progress Report

Discussion Topics

- Celebrate successes!
- Strategies for maintaining success
- Lesson learned

Experiential Exercise

- Sharing of Body Confidence Projects

Homework

- The Journey Is Just Beginning
- Use Your BC Journal Regularly or As Needed

Closing Circle

- Gratitude

About the Author

Penny Plautz is an ACE (American Council on Exercise) Certified Fitness Instructor and Creativity Coach. She is the owner of TransforMotion Studios, an exercise studio and creativity center in Illinois. She has managed health clubs in Texas and New Mexico and has served as a faculty member at Santa Fe Community College. Her books, *Wellness Works!* and *Wellness Works! For Facilitators* have been used in the Dartmouth College physical education curriculum and in other universities. Her audiotapes include *Stressed For Success* and *Creating Balance*. Her online courses include Body Confidence From The Inside Out, Secrets to Stress Less Living, Read It & Leap, and Unleash Your Creativity.

When she's not teaching or writing in Illinois, Ms. Plautz spends her time in Santa Fe, New Mexico, hiking with her dog and coaching others in the creative process.

For information on her other books and courses, visit her website at www.wellpower.com.

CPSIA information can be obtained at www.ICGtesting.com
Printed in the USA
LVOW131926010413

327049LV00001B/141/A